Vet in Harness

James Herriot grew up in Glasgow and qualified as a veterinary surgeon at Glasgow Veterinary College. Shortly afterwards he took up a position as an assistant in North Yorkshire where, with the exception of his wartime service in the RAF, he has remained. *If Only They Could Talk* and *It Shouldn't Happen to a Vet*, published in one volume with the title *All Creatures Great and Small*, has become a top American bestseller. He has also written *Let Sleeping Vets Lie*.

His interests outside his work are music and dog walking. He is married, with a son who is a veterinary surgeon and a daughter who is a doctor.

James Herriot is a pseudonym.

James Herriot
Vet in harness

Pan Books London and Sydney

First published 1974 by Michael Joseph Ltd
This edition published 1975 by Pan Books Ltd,
Cavaye Place, London SW10 9PG
2nd printing 1976
© James Herriot 1974
ISBN 0 330 24663 1
Printed and bound in Great Britain by
Cox & Wyman Ltd, London, Reading and Fakenham

With love to my mother
in dear old Glasgow town

1

As I crawled into bed and put my arm around Helen it occurred to me, not for the first time, that there are few pleasures in this world to compare with snuggling up to a nice woman when you are half frozen.

There weren't any electric blankets in the thirties. Which was a pity because nobody needed the things more than country vets. It is surprising how deeply bone-marrow cold a man can get when he is dragged from his bed in the small hours and made to strip off in farm buildings when his metabolism is at a low ebb. Often the worst part was coming back to bed; I often lay exhausted for over an hour, longing for sleep but kept awake until my icy limbs and feet had thawed out.

But since my marriage such things were but a dark memory. Helen stirred in her sleep – she had got used to her husband leaving her in the night and returning like a blast from the North Pole – and instinctively moved nearer to me. With a sigh of thankfulness I felt the blissful warmth envelop me and almost immediately the events of the last two hours began to recede into unreality.

It had started with the aggressive shrilling of the bedside phone at one a.m. And it was Sunday morning, a not unusual time for some farmers after a late Saturday night to have a look round their stock and decide to send for the vet.

This time it was Harold Ingledew. And it struck me right away that he would have just about had time to get back to his farm after his ten pints at the Four Horse Shoes where they weren't too fussy about closing time.

And there was a significant slur in the thin croak of his voice.

'I 'ave a ewe amiss. Will you come?'

'Is she very bad?' In my semi-conscious state I always clung to the faint hope that one night somebody would say it would wait till morning. It had never happened yet and it didn't happen now: Mr Ingledew was not to be denied.

'Aye, she's in a bad way. She'll have to have summat done for 'er soon.'

Not a minute to lose, I thought bitterly. But she had probably been in a bad way all the evening when Harold was out carousing.

Still, there were compensations. A sick sheep didn't present any great threat. It was worst when you had to get out of bed facing the prospect of a spell of sheer hard labour in your enfeebled state. But in this case I was confident that I would be able to adopt my half-awake technique; which meant simply that I would be able to go out there and deal with the emergency and return between the sheets while still enjoying many of the benefits of sleep.

There was so much night work in country practice that I had been compelled to perfect this system as, I suspect, had many of my fellow practitioners. I had done some sterling work while in a somnambulistic limbo.

So, eyes closed, I tiptoed across the carpet and pulled on my working clothes. I effortlessly accomplished the journey down the long flights of stairs but when I opened the side door the system began to crumble, because even in the shelter of the high-walled garden the wind struck at me with savage force. It was difficult to stay asleep. In the yard as I backed out of the garage the high branches of the elms groaned in the darkness as they bent before the blast.

Driving from the town I managed to slip back into my trance and my mind played lazily with the phenomenon of Harold Ingledew. This drinking of his was so out of character. He was a tiny mouse of a man about seventy years old and when he came into the surgery on an occasional market day it was difficult to extract more than a few muttered words from him. Dressed in his best suit, his scrawny neck protruding from a shirt collar several sizes too big for him, he was the very picture of a meek and solid citizen; the watery blue eyes and fleshless cheeks added to the effect and only the brilliant red colouration of the tip of his nose gave any hint of other possibilities.

His fellow smallholders in Therby village were all steady

characters and did not indulge beyond a social glass of beer now and then, and his next door neighbour had been somewhat bitter when he spoke to me a few weeks ago.

'He's nowt but a bloody nuisance is awd Harold.'

'How do you mean?'

'Well, every Saturday night and every market night he's up roarin' and singin' till four o'clock in the mornin'.'

'Harold Ingledew? Surely not! He's such a quiet little chap.'

'Aye, he is for the rest of t'week.'

'But I can't imagine him singing!'

'You should live next door to 'im, Mr Herriot. He makes a 'ell of a racket. There's no sleep for anybody till he settles down.'

Since then I had heard from another source that this was perfectly true and that Mrs Ingledew tolerated it because her husband was entirely submissive at all other times.

The road to Therby had a few sharp little switchbacks before it dipped to the village and looking down I could see the long row of silent houses curving away to the base of the fell which by day hung in peaceful green majesty over the huddle of roofs but now bulked black and menacing under the moon.

As I stepped from the car and hurried round to the back of the house the wind caught at me again, jerking me to wakefulness as though somebody had thrown a bucket of water over me. But for a moment I forgot the cold in the feeling of shock as the noise struck me. Singing . . . loud raucous singing echoing around the old stones of the yard.

It was coming from the lighted kitchen window.

'JUST A SONG AT TWILIGHT, WHEN THE LIGHTS ARE LOW!'

I looked inside and saw little Harold sitting with his stock-inged feet extended towards the dying embers of the fire while one hand clutched a bottle of brown ale.

'AND THE FLICKERING SHADOWS SOFTLY COME AND GO!' He was really letting it rip, head back, mouth wide.

I thumped on the kitchen door.

'THOUGH THE HEART BE WEARY, SAD THE DAY AND LONG!'

replied Harold's reedy tenor and I banged impatiently at the woodwork again.

The noise ceased and I waited an unbelievably long time till I heard the key turning and the bolt rattling back. The little man pushed his nose out and gave me a questioning look.

'I've come to see your sheep,' I said.

'Oh aye.' He nodded curtly with none of his usual diffidence. 'Ah'll put me boots on.' He banged the door in my face and I heard the bolt shooting home.

Taken aback as I was I realised that he wasn't being deliberately rude. Bolting the door was proof that he was doing everything mechanically. But for all that he had left me standing in an uncharitable spot. Vets will tell you that there are corners in farmyards which are colder than any hill top and I was in one now. Just beyond the kitchen door was a stone archway leading to the open fields and through this black opening there whistled a Siberian draught which cut effortlessly through my clothes.

I had begun to hop from one foot to the other when the singing started again.

'THERE'S AN OLD MILL BY THE STREAM, NELLIE DEAN!'

Horrified, I rushed back to the window. Harold was back in his chair, pulling on a vast boot and taking his time about it. As he bellowed he poked owlishly at the lace holes and occasionally refreshed himself from the bottle of brown ale.

I tapped on the window. 'Please hurry, Mr Ingledew.'

'WHERE WE USED TO SIT AND DREAM, NELLIE DEAN!' bawled Harold in response.

My teeth had begun to chatter before he got both boots on but at last he reappeared in the doorway.

'Come on then,' I gasped. 'Where is this ewe? Have you got her in one of these boxes?'

The old man raised his eyebrows. 'Oh, she's not 'ere.'

'Not here?'

'Nay, she's up at t'top buildings.'

'Right back up the road, you mean?'

'Aye, ah stopped off on t'way home and had a look at 'er.'

10

I stamped and rubbed my hands. 'Well, we'll have to drive back up. But there's no water, is there? You'd better bring a bucket of warm water, some soap and a towel.'

'Very good.' He nodded solemnly and before I knew what was happening the door was slammed shut and bolted and I was alone again in the darkness. I trotted immediately to the window and was not surprised to see Harold seated comfortably again. He leaned forward and lifted the kettle from the hearth and for a dreadful moment I thought he was going to start heating the water on the ashes of the fire. But with a gush of relief I saw him take hold of a ladle and reach into the primitive boiler in the old black grate.

'AND THE WATERS AS THEY FLOW SEEM TO MURMUR SWEET AND LOW!' he warbled, happy at his work, as he unhurriedly filled a bucket.

I think he had forgotten I was there when he finally came out because he looked at me blankly as he sang.

'YOU'RE MY HEART'S DESIRE, I LOVE YOU, NELLIE DEAN!' he informed me at the top of his voice.

'All right, all right,' I grunted. 'Let's go.' I hurried him into the car and we set off on the way I had come.

Harold held the bucket at an angle on his lap, and as we went over the switchbacks the water slopped gently on to my knee. The atmosphere in the car soon became so highly charged with beer fumes that I began to feel lightheaded.

'In 'ere!' the old man barked suddenly as a gate appeared in the headlights. I pulled on to the grass verge and stood on one leg for a few moments till I had shaken a surplus pint or two of water from my trousers. We went through the gate and I began to hurry towards the dark bulk of the hillside barn, but I noticed that Harold wasn't following me. He was walking aimlessly around the field.

'What are you doing, Mr Ingledew?'

'Lookin' for t'ewe.'

'You mean she's outside?' I repressed an impulse to scream.

'Aye, she lambed this afternoon and ah thowt she'd be right enough out 'ere.' He produced a torch, a typical farmer's torch

– tiny and with a moribund battery – and projected a fitful beam into the darkness. It made not the slightest difference.

As I stumbled across the field a sense of hopelessness assailed me. Above, the ragged clouds scurried across the face of the moon but down here I could see nothing. And it was so cold. The recent frosts had turned the ground to iron and the crisp grass cowered under the piercing wind. I had just decided that there was no way of finding an animal in this black waste land when Harold piped up.

'She's over 'ere.'

And sure enough when I groped my way towards the sound of his voice he was standing by an unhappy looking ewe. I don't know what instinct had brought him to her but there she was. And she was obviously in trouble; her head hung down miserably and when I put my hand on her fleece she took only a few faltering steps instead of galloping off as a healthy sheep would. Beside her, a tiny lamb huddled close to her flank.

I lifted her tail and took her temperature. It was normal. There were no signs of the usual post-lambing ailments; no staggering to indicate a deficiency, no discharge or accelerated respirations. But there was something very far wrong.

I looked again at the lamb. He was an unusually early arrival in this high country and it seemed unfair to bring the little creature into the inhospitable world of a Yorkshire March. And he was so small . . . yes . . . it was beginning to filter through to me. He was too damn small for a single lamb.

'Bring me that bucket, Mr Ingledew!' I cried. I could hardly wait to see if I was right. But as I balanced the receptacle on the grass the full horror of the situation smote me. I was going to have to strip off.

They don't give vets medals for bravery but as I pulled off my overcoat and jacket and stood shivering in my shirt sleeves on that black hillside I felt I deserved one.

'Hold her head,' I gasped and soaped my arm quickly. By the light of the torch I felt my way into the vagina and I didn't have to go very far before I found what I expected; a woolly little skull. It was bent downwards with the nose under the pelvis and the legs were back.

'There's another lamb in here,' I said. 'It's laid wrong or it would have been born with its mate this afternoon.'

Even as I spoke my fingers had righted the presentation and I drew the little creature gently out and deposited him on the grass. I hadn't expected him to be alive after his delayed entry but as he made contact with the cold ground his limbs gave a convulsive twitch and almost immediately I felt his ribs heaving under my hand.

For a moment I forgot the knife-like wind in the thrill which I always found in new life, the thrill that was always fresh, always warm. The ewe, too, seemed stimulated because in the darkness I felt her nose pushing interestedly at the new arrival.

But my pleasant ruminations were cut short by a scuffling from behind me and some muffled words.

'Bugger it!' mumbled Harold.

'What's the matter?'

'Ah've kicked bucket ower.'

'Oh no! Is the water all gone?'

'Aye, nowt left.'

Well this was great. My arm was smeared with mucus after being inside the ewe. I couldn't possibly put my jacket on without a wash.

Harold's voice issued again from the darkness. 'There's some watter ower at building.'

'Oh good. We've got to get this ewe and lambs over there anyway.' I threw my clothes over my shoulder, tucked a lamb under each arm and began to blunder over the tussocks of grass to where I thought the barn lay. The ewe, clearly feeling better without her uncomfortable burden, trotted behind me.

It was Harold again who had to give me directions.

'Ower 'ere!' he shouted.

When I reached the barn I cowered thankfully behind the massive stones. It was no night for a stroll in shirt sleeves. Shaking uncontrollably I peered at the old man. I could just see his form in the last faint radiance of the torch and I wasn't quite sure what he was doing. He had lifted a stone from the pasture and was bashing something with it; then I realised he was bending over the water trough, breaking the ice.

When he had finished he plunged the bucket into the trough and handed it to me.

'There's your watter,' he said triumphantly.

I thought I had reached the ultimate in frigidity but when I plunged my hands into the black liquid with its floating icebergs I changed my mind. The torch had finally expired and I lost the soap very quickly. When I found I was trying to work up a lather with one of the pieces of ice I gave it up and dried my arms.

Somewhere nearby I could hear Harold humming under his breath, as comfortable as if he was by his own fireside. The vast amount of alcohol surging through his bloodstream must have made him impervious to the cold.

We pushed the ewe and lambs into the barn which was piled high with hay and before leaving I struck a match and looked at the little sheep and her new family settled comfortably among the fragrant clover. They would be safe and warm in there till morning.

My journey back to the village was less hazardous because the bucket on Harold's knee was empty. I dropped him outside his house, then I had to drive to the bottom of the village to turn; and as I came past the house again the sound forced its way into the car.

'IF YOU WERE THE ONLY GIRL IN THE WORLD AND I WERE THE ONLY BOY!'

I stopped, wound the window down and listened in wonder. It was incredible how the noise reverberated around the quiet street and if it went on till four o'clock in the morning as the neighbours said, then they had my sympathy.

'NOTHING ELSE WOULD MATTER IN THE WORLD TODAY!'

It struck me suddenly that I could soon get tired of Harold's singing. His volume was impressive but for all that he would never be in great demand at Covent Garden; he constantly

14

wavered off key and there was a grating quality in his top notes which set my teeth on edge.

'WE WOULD GO ON LOVING IN THE SAME OLD WAY!'

Hurriedly I wound the window up and drove off. As the heaterless car picked its way between the endless flitting pattern of walls I crouched in frozen immobility behind the wheel. I had now reached the state of total numbness and I can't remember much about my return to the yard at Skeldale House, nor my automatic actions of putting away the car, swinging shut the creaking doors of what had once been the old coach house, and trailing slowly down the long garden.

But a realisation of my blessings began to return when I slid into bed and Helen, instead of shrinking away from me as it would have been natural to do, deliberately draped her feet and legs over the human ice block that was her husband. The bliss was unbelievable. It was worth getting out just to come back to this.

I glanced at the luminous dial of the alarm clock. It was three o'clock and as the warmth flowed over me and I drifted away, my mind went back to the ewe and lambs, snug in their scented barn. They would be asleep now, I would soon be asleep, everybody would be asleep.

Except, that is, Harold Ingledew's neighbours. They still had an hour to go.

2

I had only to sit up in bed to look right across Darrowby to the hills beyond.

I got up and walked to the window. It was going to be a fine morning and the early sun glanced over the weathered reds and greys of the jumbled roofs, some of them sagging under their

15

burden of ancient tiles, and brightened the tufts of green where trees pushed upwards from the gardens among the bristle of chimney pots. And behind everything the calm bulk of the fells.

It was my good fortune that this was the first thing I saw every morning; after Helen, of course, which was better still.

Following our unorthodox tuberculin testing honeymoon we had set up our first home on the top of Skeldale House. Siegfried, my boss up to my wedding and now my partner, had offered us free use of these empty rooms on the third storey and we had gratefully accepted; and though it was a makeshift arrangement there was an airy charm, an exhilaration in our high perch that many would have envied.

It was makeshift because everything at that time had a temporary complexion and we had no idea how long we would be there. Siegfried and I had both volunteered for the R.A.F. and were on deferred service but that is all I am going to say about the war. This book is not about such things which in any case were so very far from Darrowby; it is the story of the months I had with Helen between our marriage and my call-up and is about the ordinary things which have always made up our lives; my work, the animals, the Dales.

This front room was our bed-sitter and though it was not luxuriously furnished it did have an excellent bed, a carpet, a handsome side table which had belonged to Helen's mother and two armchairs. It had an ancient wardrobe, too, but the lock didn't work and the only way we kept the door closed was by jamming one of my socks in it. The toe always dangled outside but it never seemed of any importance.

I went out and across a few feet of landing to our kitchen-dining room at the back. This apartment was definitely spartan. I clumped over bare boards to a bench we had rigged against the wall by the window. This held a gas ring and our crockery and cutlery. I seized a tall jug and began my long descent to the main kitchen downstairs because one minor snag was that there was no water at the top of the house. Down two flights to the three rooms on the first storey then down two more and a final gallop along the passage to the big stone-flagged kitchen at the end.

I filled the jug and returned to our eyrie two steps at a time. I wouldn't like to do this now whenever I needed water but at that time I didn't find it the least inconvenience.

Helen soon had the kettle boiling and we drank our first cup of tea by the window looking down on the long garden. From up here we had an aerial view of the unkempt lawns, the fruit trees, the wistaria climbing the weathered brick towards our window, and the high walls with their old stone copings stretching away to the cobbled yard under the elms. Every day I went up and down that path to the garage in the yard but it looked so different from above.

'Wait a minute, Helen,' I said. 'Let me sit on that chair.'

She had laid the breakfast on the bench where we ate and this was where the difficulty arose. Because it was a tall bench and our recently acquired high stool fitted it but our chair didn't.

'No, I'm all right, Jim, really I am.' She smiled at me reassuringly from her absurd position, almost at eye level with her plate.

'You can't be all right,' I retorted. 'Your chin's nearly in among your cornflakes. Please let me sit there.'

She patted the seat of the stool. 'Come on, stop arguing. Sit down and have your breakfast.'

This, I felt, just wouldn't do. I tried a different tack.

'Helen!' I said severely. 'Get off that chair!'

'No!' she replied without looking at me, her lips pushed forward in a characteristic pout which I always found enchanting but which also meant she wasn't kidding.

I was at a loss. I toyed with the idea of pulling her off the chair, but she was a big girl. We had had a previous physical try-out when a minor disagreement had escalated into a wrestling match and though I thoroughly enjoyed the contest and actually won in the end I had been surprised by her sheer strength. At this time in the morning I didn't feel up to it. I sat on the stool.

17

After breakfast Helen began to boil water for the washing-up, the next stage in our routine. Meanwhile I went downstairs, collected my gear, including suture material for a foal which had cut its leg and went out the side door into the garden. Just about opposite the rockery I turned and looked up at our window. It was open at the bottom and an arm emerged holding a dishcloth. I waved and the dishcloth waved back furiously. It was the start to every day.

And, driving from the yard, it seemed a good start. In fact everything was good. The raucous cawing of the rooks in the elms above as I closed the double doors, the clean fragrance of the air which greeted me every morning, and the challenge and interest of my job.

The injured foal was at Robert Corner's farm and I hadn't been there long before I spotted Jock, his sheepdog. And I began to watch the dog because behind a vet's daily chore of treating his patients there is always the fascinating kaleidoscope of animal personality and Jock was an interesting case.

A lot of farm dogs are partial to a little light relief from their work. They like to play and one of their favourite games is chasing cars off the premises. Often I drove off with a hairy form galloping alongside and the dog would usually give a final defiant bark after a few hundred yards to speed me on my way. But Jock was different.

He was really dedicated. Car chasing to him was a deadly serious art which he practised daily without a trace of levity. Corner's farm was at the end of a long track, twisting for nearly a mile between its stone walls down through the gently sloping fields to the road below and Jock didn't consider he had done his job properly until he had escorted his chosen vehicle right to the very foot. So his hobby was an exacting one.

I watched him now as I finished stitching the foal's leg and began to tie on a bandage. He was slinking about the buildings, a skinny little creature who, without his mass of black and white hair would have been an almost invisible mite, and he was playing out a transparent charade of pretending he was taking no notice of me – wasn't the least bit interested in my presence, in fact. But his furtive glances in the direction of the stable, his repeated criss-crossing of my line of vision gave him away. He was waiting for his big moment.

When I was putting on my shoes and throwing my wellingtons into the boot I saw him again. Or rather part of him; just a long nose and one eye protruding from beneath a broken door. It wasn't till I had started the engine and begun to move off that he finally declared himself, stealing out from his hiding place, body low, tail trailing, eyes fixed intently on the car's front wheels, and as I gathered speed and headed down the track he broke into an effortless lope.

I had been through this before and was always afraid he might run in front of me so I put my foot down and began to hurtle downhill. This was where Jock came into his own. I often wondered how he'd fare against a racing greyhound because by golly he could run. That sparse frame housed a perfect physical machine and the slender limbs reached and flew again and again, devouring the stony ground beneath, keeping up with the speeding car with joyful ease.

There was a sharp bend about half way down and here Jock invariably sailed over the wall and streaked across the turf, a little dark blur against the green, and having craftily cut off the corner he reappeared like a missile zooming over the grey stones lower down. This put him into a nice position for the run to the road and when he finally saw me on to the tarmac my last view of him was of a happy panting face looking after me. Clearly he considered it was a job well done and he would wander contentedly back up to the farm to await the next session, perhaps with the postman or the baker's van.

And there was another side to Jock. He was an outstanding performer at the sheepdog trials and Mr Corner had won many trophies with him. In fact the farmer could have sold the little animal for a lot of money but couldn't be persuaded to part with him. Instead he purchased a bitch, a scrawny little female counterpart of Jock and a trial winner in her own right. With this combination Mr Corner thought he could breed some world-beating types for sale. On my visits to the farm the bitch joined in the car-chasing but it seemed as though she was doing it more or less to humour her new mate and she always gave up at the first bend leaving Jock in command. You could see her heart wasn't in it.

When the pups arrived, seven fluffy black balls tumbling about the yard and getting under everybody's feet, Jock watched indulgently as they tried to follow him in his pursuit of my vehicle and you could almost see him laughing as they fell over their feet and were left trailing far behind.

It happened that I didn't have to go there for about ten months but I saw Robert Corner in the market occasionally and he told me he was training the pups and they were shaping well. Not that they needed much training; it was in their blood and he said they had tried to round up the cattle and sheep nearly as soon as they could walk. When I finally saw them they were like seven Jocks – meagre, darting little creatures flitting noiselessly about the buildings – and it didn't take me long to find out that they had learned more than sheep herding from their father. There was something very evocative about the way they began to prowl around in the background as I prepared to get into my car, peeping furtively from behind straw bales, slinking with elaborate nonchalance into favourable positions for a quick getaway. And as I settled in my seat I could sense they were all crouched in readiness for the off.

I revved my engine, let in the clutch with a bump and shot across the yard and in a second the immediate vicinity erupted in a mass of hairy forms. I roared on to the track and put my foot down and on either side of me the little animals pelted along shoulder to shoulder, their faces all wearing the intent fanatical expression I knew so well. When Jock cleared the wall the seven pups went with him and when they reappeared and entered the home straight I noticed something different. On past occasions Jock had always had one eye on the car – this was what he considered his opponent; but now on that last quarter mile as he hurtled along at the head of a shaggy phalanx he was glancing at the pups on either side as though they were the main opposition.

And there was no doubt he was in trouble. Superbly fit though he was, these stringy bundles of bone and sinew which he had fathered had all his speed plus the newly minted energy of youth and it was taking every shred of his power to keep up with them. Indeed there was one terrible moment when he stumbled and was engulfed by the bounding creatures around him; it seemed that all was lost but there was a core of steel in Jock. Eyes popping, nostrils dilated, he fought his way through the pack until by the time we reached the road he was once more in the lead.

But it had taken its toll. I slowed down before driving away and looked down at the little animal standing with lolling tongue and heaving flanks on the grass verge. It must have been like this with all the other vehicles and it wasn't a merry game any more. I suppose it sounds silly to say you could read a dog's thoughts but everything in his posture betrayed the mounting apprehension that his days of supremacy were numbered. Just round the corner lay the unthinkable ignominy of being left trailing in the rear of that litter of young upstarts and as I drew away Jock looked after me and his expression was eloquent.

'How long can I keep this up?'

I felt for the little dog and on my next visit to the farm about two months later I wasn't looking forward to witnessing the final degradation which I felt was inevitable. But when I drove into the yard I found the place strangely unpopulated.

Robert Corner was forking hay into the cow's racks in the byre. He turned as I came in.

'Where are all your dogs?' I asked.

He put down his fork. 'All gone. By gaw, there's a market for good workin' sheepdogs. I've done right well out of t'job.'

'But you've still got Jock?'

'Oh aye, ah couldn't part with t'awd lad. He's over there.'

And so he was, creeping around as of old, pretending he wasn't watching me. And when the happy time finally arrived and I drove away it was like it used to be with the lean little animal haring along by the side of the car, but relaxed, enjoying the game, winging effortlessly over the wall and beating the car down to the tarmac with no trouble at all.

I think I was as relieved as he was that he was left alone with his supremacy unchallenged; that he was still top dog.

3

You could hardly expect to find a more unlikely character in Darrowby than Roland Partridge. The thought came to me for the hundredth time as I saw him peering through the window which looked on to Trengate just a little way up the other side of the street from our surgery.

He was tapping the glass and beckoning to me and the eyes behind the thick spectacles were wide with concern. I waited and when he opened the door I stepped straight from the street into his living room because these were tiny dwellings with only a kitchen in the rear and a single small bedroom overlooking the street above. But when I went in I had the familiar feeling of surprise. Because most of the other occupants of the row were farmworkers and their furnishings were orthodox; but this place was a studio.

An easel stood in the light from the window and the walls were covered from floor to ceiling with paintings. Unframed canvases were stacked everywhere and the few ornate chairs and the table with its load of painted china and other bric-à-brac added to the artistic atmosphere.

The simple explanation was, of course, that Mr Partridge was in fact an artist. But the unlikely aspect came into it when you learned that this middle-aged velvet-jacketed aesthete was the son of a small farmer, a man whose forebears had been steeped in the soil for generations.

'I happened to see you passing there, Mr Herriot,' he said. 'Are you terribly busy?'

'Not too busy, Mr Partridge. Can I help you?'

He nodded gravely. 'I wonder whether you could spare a moment to look at Percy. I'd be most grateful.'

'Of course,' I replied. 'Where is he?'

He was ushering me towards the kitchen when there was a bang on the outer door and Bert Hardisty the postman burst in. Bert was a rough-hewn character and he dumped a parcel unceremoniously on the table.

'There y'are, Rolie!' he shouted and turned to go.

Mr Partridge gazed with unruffled dignity at the retreating back. 'Thank you very much indeed, Bertram, good day to you.'

Here was another thing. The postman and the artist were both Darrowby born and bred, had the same social background, had gone to the same school, yet their voices were quite different. Roland Partridge, in fact, spoke with the precise, well-modulated syllables of a barrister-at-law.

We went into the kitchen. This was where he cooked for himself in his bachelor state. When his father died many years ago he had sold the farm immediately. Apparently his whole nature was appalled by the earthy farming scene and he could not get out quickly enough. At any rate he had got sufficient money from the sale to indulge his interests and he had taken up painting and lived ever since in this humble cottage, resolutely doing his own thing. This had all happened long before I came to Darrowby and the dangling lank hair was silver now. I always had the feeling that he was happy in his way because I couldn't imagine that small, rather exquisite figure plodding round a muddy farmyard.

It was probably in keeping with his nature that he had never married. There was a touch of asceticism in the thin cheeks and pale blue eyes and it was possible that this self-contained imperturbable personality might denote a lack of warmth. But that didn't hold good with regard to his dog, Percy.

He loved Percy with a fierce protective passion and as the

little animal trotted towards him he bent over him, his face alight with tenderness.

'He looks pretty bright to me,' I said. 'He's not sick, is he?'

'No...no...' Mr Partridge seemed strangely ill at ease. 'He's perfectly well in himself, but I want you to look at him and see if you notice anything.'

I looked. And I saw only what I had always seen, the snow-white, shaggy-haired little object regarded by local dog breeders and other *cognoscenti* as a negligible mongrel but nevertheless one of my favourite patients. Mr Partridge, looking through the window of a pet shop in Brawton about five years ago had succumbed immediately to the charms of two soulful eyes gazing up at him from a six-week-old tangle of white hair and had put down his five bob and rushed the little creature home. Percy had been described in the shop somewhat vaguely as a 'terrier' and Mr Partridge had flirted fearfully with the idea of having his tail docked; but such was his infatuation that he couldn't bring himself to cause such a mutilation and the tail had grown in a great fringed curve almost full circle over the back.

To me, the tail nicely balanced the head which was undoubtedly a little too big for the body but Mr Partridge had been made to suffer for it. His old friends in Darrowby who, like all country folks, considered themselves experts with animals, were free with their comments. I had heard them at it. When Percy was young it was:

'Time ye had that tail off, Rolie. Ah'll bite it off for ye if ye like.' And later, again and again. 'Hey Rolie, you should've had that dog's tail off when he were a pup. He looks bloody daft like that.'

When asked Percy's breed Mr Partridge always replied haughtily, 'Sealyham Cross', but it wasn't as simple as that; the tiny body with its luxuriant bristling coat, the large, rather noble head with high, pricked ears, the short, knock-kneed legs and that tail made him a baffling mixture.

Mr Partridge's friends again were merciless, referring to Percy as a 'tripe-'ound' or a 'mouse-'ound' and though the little artist received these railleries with a thin smile I knew they bit deep. He had a high regard for me based simply on the fact that the first time I saw Percy I exclaimed quite spontaneously, 'What a beautiful little dog!' And since I have never had much time for the points and fads of dog breeding I really meant it.

'Just what is wrong, Mr Partridge ?' I asked. 'I can't see anything unusual.'

Again the little man appeared to be uneasy. 'Well now, watch as he walks across the floor. Come, Percy my dear.' He moved away from me and the dog followed him.

'No . . . no . . . I don't quite understand what you mean.'

'Watch again.' He set off once more. 'It's at his . . . his er . . . back end.'

I crouched down. 'Ah now, yes, wait a minute. Just hold him there, will you ?'

I went over and had a close look. 'I see it now. One of his testicles is slightly enlarged.'

'Yes . . . yes . . . quite.' Mr Partridge's face turned a shade pinker. 'That is . . . er . . . what I thought.'

'Hang on to him a second while I examine it.' I lifted the scrotum and palpated gently. 'Yes, the left one is definitely bigger and it is harder too.'

'Is it . . . anything serious ?'

I paused. 'No, I shouldn't think so. Tumours of the testicles are not uncommon in dogs and fortunately they aren't inclined to metastasise – spread through the body – very readily. So I shouldn't worry too much.'

I added the last bit hastily because at the mention of the word 'tumour' the colour had drained from his face alarmingly.

'That's a growth, isn't it ?' he stammered.

'Yes, but there are all kinds and a lot of them are not malignant. So don't worry but please keep an eye on him. It may not grow much but if it does you must let me know immediately.'

'I see . . . and if it does grow ?'

'Well the only thing would be to remove the testicle.'

'An operation ?' The little man stared at me and for a moment I thought he would faint.

'Yes, but not a serious one. Quite straightforward, really.' I bent down and felt the enlargement again. It was very slight. From the front end, Percy kept up a continuous musical growling. I grinned. He always did that – when I took his temperature, cut his nails, anything; a nonstop grumble and it didn't mean a thing. I knew him well enough to realise there was no viciousness in him; he was merely asserting his virility, reminding me what a tough fellow he was, and it was not idle boasting because for all his lack of size he was a proud, mettlesome little dog, absolutely crammed with character.

After I had left the house I looked back and saw Mr Partridge standing there watching me. He was clasping and unclasping his hands.

And even when I was back in the surgery half of me was still in that odd little studio. I had to admire Mr Partridge for doing exactly what he wanted to do because in Darrowby he would never get any credit for it. A good horseman or cricketer would be revered in the town but an artist . . . never. Not even if he became famous, and Mr Partridge would never be famous. A few people bought his paintings but he could not have lived on the proceeds. I had one of them hanging in our bed-sitter and to my mind he had a definite gift. In fact I would have tried to afford more of them but for the fact that he obviously shrank from that aspect of the Yorkshire Dales which I loved most.

If I had been able to paint I would have wanted to show how the walls climbed everywhere over the stark fell-sides. I would have tried to capture the magic of the endless empty moors with the reeds trembling over the black bog pools. But Mr Partridge went only for the cosy things; willows hanging by a rustic bridge, village churches, rose-covered cottages.

Since Percy was a near neighbour I saw him nearly every day, either from our bed-sitter at the top of the house or from the surgery below. His master exercised him with great zeal and regularity and it was a common sight to see the artist passing on the other side of the road with the little animal trotting proudly beside him. But from that distance it was impossible to see if the tumour was progressing, and since I heard nothing from Mr Partridge I assumed that all was well. Maybe that thing had grown no more. Sometimes it happened that way.

Keeping a close watch on the little dog reminded me of other incidents connected with him, particularly the number of times he was involved in a fight. Not that Percy ever started a brawl – at ten inches high he wasn't stupid enough for that – but somehow big dogs when they saw that dainty white figure prancing along were inclined to go for him on sight. I witnessed some of these attacks from our windows and the same thing happened every time; a quick flurry of limbs, a snarling and yelping and then the big dog retreated bleeding.

Percy never had a mark on him – that tremendous thick coat gave him complete protection – but he always got a nip in from underneath. I had stitched up several of the local street fighters after Percy had finished with them.

It must have been about six weeks later when Mr Partridge came in again. He looked tense.

'I'd like you to have a look at Percy again, Mr Herriot.'

I lifted the dog on to the surgery table and I didn't need to examine him very closely.

'It's quite a lot bigger, I'm afraid.' I looked across the table at the little man.

'Yes, I know.' He hesitated. 'What do you suggest?'

'Oh there's no doubt at all he'll have to come in for an operation. That thing must come off.'

Horror and despair flickered behind the thick spectacles.

'An operation!' He leaned on the table with both hands.

'I hate the idea, I just can't bear the thought of it!'

I smiled reassuringly. 'I know how you feel, but honestly there's nothing to worry about. As I told you before, it's quite a simple procedure.'

'Oh I know, I know,' he moaned. 'But I don't want him to be . . . cut about, you understand . . . it's just the idea of it.'

And I couldn't persuade him. He remained adamant and marched resolutely from the surgery with his pet. I watched him crossing the road to his house and I knew he had let himself in for a load of worry, but I didn't realise just how bad it was going to be.

It was to be a kind of martyrdom.

4

I do not think martyrdom is too strong a word for what Mr Partridge went through over the next few weeks, because with the passage of time that testicle became more and more massive and due to the way Percy carried his tail the thing was lamentably conspicuous.

People used to turn and stare as man and dog made their way down the street, Percy trotting bravely, his master, eyes rigidly to the front, putting up a magnificent pretence of being quite unaware of anything unusual. It really hurt me to see them and I found the sight of the smart little dog's disfigurement particularly hard to bear.

Mr Partridge's superior facade had always made him a natural target for a certain amount of legpulling which he bore stoically; but the fact that it now involved his pet pierced him to the soul.

One afternoon he brought him over to the surgery and I could see that the little man was almost in tears. Gloomily I examined the offending organ which was now about six inches long; gross, pendulous, undeniably ludicrous.

'You know, Mr Herriot,' the artist gasped. 'Some boys chalked on my window, "Roll up and see the famous Chinese dog, Wun Hung Lo." I've just been wiping it off.'

I rubbed my chin. 'Well that's an ancient joke, Mr Partridge. I shouldn't worry about that.'

'But I do worry! I can't sleep because of the thing!'

'For heaven's sake, then, why don't you let me operate? I could put the whole business right for you.'

'No! No! I can't do that!' His head rolled on his shoulders; he was the very picture of misery as he stared at me. 'I'm frightened, that's what it is. I'm frightened he'll die under the anaesthetic.'

'Oh come now! He's a strong little animal. There's no reason at all for such fears.'

'But there is a risk, isn't there?'

I looked at him helplessly. 'Well there's a slight risk in all operations if you come right down to it, but honestly in this case . . .'

'No! That's enough. I won't hear of it,' he burst out and seizing Percy's lead he strode away.

Things went from bad to worse after that. The tumour grew steadily, easily visible now from my vantage point in the surgery window as the dog went by on the other side of the street, and I could see too that the stares and occasional ridicule were beginning to tell on Mr Partridge. His cheeks had hollowed and he had lost some of his high colour.

But I didn't have words with him till one market day several weeks later. It was early afternoon – the time the farmers often came in to pay their bills. I was showing one of them out when I saw Percy and his master coming out of the house. And I noticed immediately that the little animal now had to swing one leg slightly to clear the massive obstruction.

On an impulse I called out and beckoned to Mr Partridge.

'Look,' I said as he came across to me. 'You've just got to let me take that thing off. It's interfering with his walking – making him lame. He can't go on like this.'

The artist didn't say anything but stared back at me with hunted eyes. We were standing there in silence when Bill Dalton came round the corner and marched up to the surgery steps, cheque book in hand. Bill was a large beefy farmer who spent most of market day in the bar of the Black Swan and he was preceded by an almost palpable wave of beer fumes.

'Nah then, Rolie lad, how ista?' he roared, slapping the little man violently on the back.

'I am quite well, William, thank you, and how are you?'

But Bill didn't answer. His attention was all on Percy who had strolled a few paces along the pavement. He watched him intently for a few moments then, repressing a giggle, he turned back to Mr Partridge with a mock-serious expression.

'Tha knows, Rolie,' he said, 'that blood 'ound of your reminds me of the young man of Devizes, whose balls were of different sizes. The one was so small it was no ball at all, but the other one won several prizes.' He finished with a shout of laughter which went on and on till he collapsed weakly against the iron railings.

For a moment I thought Mr Partridge was going to strike him. He glared up at the big man and his chin and mouth trembled with rage, then he seemed to gain control of himself and turned to me.

'Can I have a word with you, Mr Herriot?'

'Certainly.' I walked a few yards with him down the street.

'You're right,' he said. 'Percy will have to have that operation. When can you do him?'

'Tomorrow,' I replied. 'Don't give him any more food and bring him in at two in the afternoon.'

It was with a feeling of intense relief that I saw the little dog stretched on the table the next day. With Tristan as anaesthetist I quickly removed the huge testicle, going well up the spermatic cord to ensure the complete excision of all tumour tissue. The only thing which troubled me was that the scrotum itself had become involved due to the long delay in operating. This is the sort of thing that can lead to a recurrence and as I carefully cut away the affected parts of the scrotal wall I cursed Mr Partridge's procrastination. I put in the last stitch with my fingers crossed.

The little man was in such transports of joy at seeing his pet alive after my efforts and rid of that horrid excrescence that I didn't want to spoil everything by voicing my doubts; but I wasn't entirely happy. If the tumour did recur I wasn't sure just what I could do about it.

But in the meantime I enjoyed my own share of pleasure at my patient's return to normality. I felt a warm rush of satisfaction whenever I saw him tripping along, perky as ever and free from the disfigurement which had bulked so large in his master's life. Occasionally I used to stroll casually behind him on the way down Trengate into the market place, saying nothing to Mr Partridge but shooting some sharp glances at the region beneath Percy's tail.

In the meantime I had sent the removed organ off to the pathology department at Glasgow Veterinary College and their report told me that it was a Sertoli Cell Tumour. They also added the comforting information that this type was usually benign and that metastasis into the internal organs occurred in only a very small proportion of cases. Maybe this lulled me into a deeper security than was warranted because I stopped following Percy around and in fact, in the nonstop rush of new cases, forgot all about his spell of trouble.

So that when Mr Partridge brought him round to the surgery I thought it was for something else and when his master lifted him on to the table and turned him round to show his rear end I stared uncomprehendingly for a moment. But I leaned forward anxiously when I spotted the ugly swelling on the left side of the scrotum. I palpated quickly, with Percy's growls and grousings providing an irritable obbligato, and there was no doubt about it, the tumour was growing again. It meant business, too, because it was red, angry-looking, painful; a dangerously active growth if ever I had seen one.

'It's come up quite quickly, has it?' I asked.

Mr Partridge nodded. 'Yes, indeed. I can almost see it getting bigger every day.'

We were in trouble. There was no hope of trying to cut this lot away; it was a great diffuse mass without clear boundaries and I wouldn't have known where to start. Anyway, if I began any more poking about it would be just what was needed to start a spread into the internal organs, and that would be the end of Percy.

'It's worse this time, isn't it?' The little man looked at me and gulped.

'Yes . . . yes . . . I'm afraid so.'

31

'Is there anything at all you can do about it?' he asked.

I was trying to think of a painless way of telling him that there wasn't when I remembered something I had read in the Veterinary Record a week ago. It was about a new drug, Stilboestrol, which had just come out and was supposed to be useful for hormonal therapy in animals; but the bit I was thinking about was a small print extract which said it had been useful in cancer of the prostate in men. I wondered . . .

'There's one thing I'd like to try,' I said, suddenly brisk, 'I can't guarantee anything, of course, because it's something new. But we'll see what a week or two's course does.'

'Oh good, good,' Mr Partridge breathed, snatching gratefully at the straw.

I rang May and Baker's and they sent the Stilboestrol to me immediately.

I injected Percy with 10 mg of the oily suspension and put him on to 10 mg tablets daily. They were big doses for a little dog but in a desperate situation I felt they were justified. Then I sat back and waited.

For about a week the tumour continued to grow and I nearly stopped the treatment, then there was a spell lasting several days during which I couldn't be sure; but then with a surge of relief I realised there could be no further doubt – the thing wasn't getting any bigger. I wasn't going to throw my hat in the air and I knew anything could still happen but I had done something with my treatment; I had halted that fateful progress.

The artist's step acquired a fresh spring as he passed on his daily walk and then as the ugly mass actually began to diminish he would wave towards the surgery window and point happily at the little white animal trotting by his side.

Poor Mr Partridge. He was on the crest of the wave but just ahead of him was the second and more bizarre phase of his martyrdom.

At first neither I nor anybody else realised what was going on. All we knew was there suddenly seemed to be a lot of dogs in Trengate – dogs we didn't usually see, from other parts of the town; big ones, small ones, shaggy mongrels and sleek aristocrats all hanging around apparently aimlessly, but then it was noticed that there was a focal point of attraction. It was Mr Partridge's house.

And it hit me blindingly one morning as I looked out of our bedroom window. They were after Percy. For some reason he had taken on the attributes of a bitch in heat. I hurried downstairs and got out my pathology book. Yes, there it was. The Sertoli Cell tumour occasionally made dogs attractive to other male dogs. But why should it be happening now when the thing was reducing and not when it was at its height? Or could it be the Stilboestrol? The new drug was said to have a feminising effect, but surely not to that extent.

Anyway, whatever the cause, the undeniable fact remained that Percy was under siege, and as the word got around the pack increased, being augmented by several of the nearby farm dogs, a Great Dane who had made the journey from Houlton, and Magnus, the little dachshund from the Drovers' Arms. The queue started forming almost at first light and by ten o'clock there would be a milling throng almost blocking the street. Apart from the regulars the odd canine visitor passing through would join the company, and no matter what his breed or size he was readily accepted into the club, adding one more to the assortment of stupid expressions, lolling tongues and waving tails; because, motley crew though they were, they were all happily united in the roisterous, bawdy camaraderie of lust.

The strain on Mr Partridge must have been almost intolerable. At times I noticed the thick spectacles glinting balefully at the mob through his window but most of the time he kept himself in hand, working calmly at his easel as though he were oblivious that every one of the creatures outside had evil designs on his treasure.

Only rarely did his control snap. I witnessed one of these occasions when he rushed screaming from his doorway, laying about him with a walking stick; and I noticed that the polished veneer slipped from him and his cries rang out in broadest Yorkshire.

'Gerrout, ye bloody rotten buggers! Gerrout of it!'

He might as well have saved his energy because the pack scattered only for a few seconds before taking up their stations again.

I felt for the little man but there was nothing I could do about it. My main feeling was of relief that the tumour was going down but I had to admit to a certain morbid fascination at the train of events across the street.

Percy's walks were fraught with peril. Mr Partridge always armed himself with his stick before venturing from the house and kept Percy on a short lead, but his precautions were unavailing as the wave of dogs swept down on him. The besotted creatures, mad with passion, leapt on top of the little animal as the artist beat vainly on the shaggy backs and yelled at them; and the humiliating procession usually continued right across the market place to the great amusement of the inhabitants.

At lunch time most of the dogs took a break and at nightfall they all went home to bed, but there was one little brown spaniel type who, with the greatest dedication, never left his post. I think he must have gone almost without food for about two weeks because he dwindled practically to a skeleton and I think he might have died if Helen hadn't taken pieces of meat over to him when she saw him huddled trembling in the doorway in the cold darkness of the evening. I know he stayed there all night because every now and then a shrill yelping wakened me in the small hours and I deduced that Mr Partridge had got home on him with some missile from his bedroom window. But it made no difference; he continued his vigil undaunted.

I don't quite know how Mr Partridge would have survived if this state of affairs had continued indefinitely; I think his reason might have given way. But mercifully signs began to appear that the nightmare was on the wane. The mob began to thin as Percy's condition improved and one day even the little brown dog reluctantly left his beat and slunk away to his unknown home.

That was the very day I had Percy on the table for the last time. I felt a thrill of satisfaction as I ran a fold of the scrotal skin between my fingers.

'There's nothing there now, Mr Partridge. No thickening, even. Not a thing.'

The little man nodded. 'Yes, it's a miracle, isn't it! I'm very grateful to you for all you've done. I've been so terribly worried.'

'Oh, I can imagine. You've been through a bad time. But I'm really as pleased as you are yourself – it's one of the most satisfying things in practice when an experiment like this comes off.'

But often over the subsequent years, as I watched dog and master pass our window, Mr Partridge with all his dignity restored, Percy as trim and proud as ever, I wondered about that strange interlude.

Did the Stilboestrol really reduce that tumour or did it regress naturally? And were the extraordinary events caused by the treatment or the condition or both?

I could never be quite sure of the answer, but of the outcome I could be happily certain. That unpleasant growth never came back . . . and neither did all those dogs.

5

This was the real Yorkshire with the clean limestone wall riding the hill's edge and the path cutting brilliant green through the crowding heather. And, walking face on to the scented breeze I felt the old tingle of wonder at being alone on the wide moorland where nothing stirred and the spreading miles of purple blossom and green turf reached away till it met the hazy blue of the sky.

But I wasn't really alone. There was Sam, and he made all the difference. Helen had brought a lot of things into my life and Sam was one of the most precious; he was a Beagle and her own personal pet. He would be about two years old when I first saw him and I had no way of knowing that he was to be my faithful companion, my car dog, my friend who sat by my side through the lonely hours of driving till his life ended at the age of fourteen. He was the first of a series of cherished dogs whose comradeship have warmed and lightened my working life.

Sam adopted me on sight. It was as though he had read the *Faithful Hound Manual* because he was always near me; paws on the dash as he gazed eagerly through the windscreen on my rounds, head resting on my foot in our bed-sitting room, trotting just behind me wherever I moved. If I had a beer in a pub he would be under my chair and even when I was having a haircut you only had to lift the white sheet to see Sam crouching beneath my legs. The only place I didn't dare take him was to the cinema and on these occasions he crawled under the bed and sulked.

Most dogs love car riding but to Sam it was a passion which never waned – even in the night hours; he would gladly leave his basket when the world was asleep, stretch a couple of times and follow me out into the cold. He would be on to the seat before I got the car door fully open and this action became so much a part of my life that for a long time after his death I still held the door open unthinkingly, waiting for him. And I still remember the pain I felt when he did not bound inside.

And having him with me added so much to the intermissions I granted myself on my daily rounds. Whereas in offices and factories they had tea breaks I just stopped the car and stepped out into the splendour which was always at hand and walked for a spell down hidden lanes, through woods, or as today, along one of the grassy tracks which ran over the high tops.

This thing which I had always done had a new meaning now. Anybody who has ever walked a dog knows the abiding satisfaction which comes from giving pleasure to a loved animal, and the sight of the little form trotting ahead of me lent a depth which had been missing before.

Round the curve of the path I came to where the tide of heather lapped thickly down the hillside on a little slope facing invitingly into the sun. It was a call I could never resist. I looked at my watch; oh I had a few minutes to spare and there was nothing urgent ahead, just Mr Dacre's tuberculin test. In a moment I was stretched out on the springy stems, the most wonderful natural mattress in the world.

Lying there, eyes half closed against the sun's glare, the heavy heather fragrance around me, I could see the cloud shadows racing across the flanks of the fells, throwing the gulleys and crevices into momentary gloom but trailing a fresh flaring green in their wake.

Those were the days when I was most grateful I was in country practice; the shirt sleeve days when the bleak menace of the bald heights melted into friendliness, when I felt at one with all the airy life and growth about me and was glad that I had become what I never thought I would be, a doctor of farm animals.

My partner, Siegfried, would be somewhere out there, thrashing round the practice and Tristan his student brother would probably be studying in Skeldale House. This latter was quite a thought because I had never seen Tristan open a text book until lately. He had been blessed with the kind of brain which made swotting irrelevant but he would take his finals this year and even he had to get down to it. I had little doubt he would soon be a qualified man and in a way it seemed a shame that his free spirit should be shackled by the realities of veterinary practice. It would be the end of a luminous chapter.

A long-eared head blotted out the sunshine as Sam came and sat on my chest. He looked at me questioningly. He didn't hold with this laziness but I knew if I didn't move after a few minutes he would curl up philosophically on my ribs and have a sleep until I was ready to go. But this time I answered the unspoken appeal by sitting up and he leaped around me in delight as I rose and began to make my way back to the car and Mr Dacre's test.

'Move over, Bill!' Mr Dacre cried some time later as he tweaked the big bull's tail.

Nearly every farmer kept a bull in those days and they were all called Billy or Bill. I suppose it was because this was a very mature animal that he received the adult version. Being a docile beast he responded to the touch on his tail by shuffling his great bulk to one side, leaving me enough space to push in between him and the wooden partition against which he was tied by a chain.

I was reading a tuberculin test and all I wanted to do was to measure the intradermal reaction. I had to open my calipers very wide to take in the thickness of the skin on the enormous neck.

'Thirty,' I called out to the farmer.

He wrote the figure down on the testing book and laughed. 'By heck, he's got some pelt on 'im.'

'Yes,' I said, beginning to squeeze my way out. 'But he's a big fellow, isn't he?'

Just how big he was was brought home to me immediately because the bull suddenly swung round, pinning me against the partition. Cows did this regularly and I moved them by bracing my back against whatever was behind me and pushing them away. But it was different with Bill.

Gasping, I pushed with all my strength against the rolls of fat which covered the vast roan-coloured flank, but I might as well have tried to shift a house.

The farmer dropped his book and seized the tail again but this time the bull showed no response. There was no malice in his behaviour – he was simply having a comfortable lean against the boards and I don't suppose he even noticed the morsel of puny humanity wriggling frantically against his rib-cage.

Still, whether he meant it or not, the end result was the same; I was having the life crushed out of me. Pop-eyed, groaning, scarcely able to breathe, I struggled with everything I had, but I couldn't move an inch. And just when I thought things couldn't get any worse, Bill started to rub himself up and down against the partition. So that was what he had come round for; he had an itch and he just wanted to scratch it.

The effect on me was catastrophic. I was certain my internal organs were being steadily ground to pulp and as I thrashed about in complete panic the huge animal leaned even more heavily.

38

I don't like to think what would have happened if the wood behind me had not been old and rotten, but just as I felt my senses leaving me there was a cracking and splintering and I fell through into the next stall. Lying there like a stranded fish on a bed of shattered timbers I looked up at Mr Dacre, waiting till my lungs started to work again.

The farmer, having got over his first alarm, was rubbing his upper lip vigorously in a polite attempt to stop himself laughing. His little girl who had watched the whole thing from her vantage point in one of the hay racks had no such inhibitions. Screaming with delight, she pointed at me.

'Ooo, Dad, Dad, look at that man! Did you see him, Dad, did you see him? Ooo what a funny man!' She went into helpless convulsions. She was only about five but I had a feeling she would remember my performance all her life.

At length I picked myself up and managed to brush the matter off lightly, but after I had driven a mile or so from the farm I stopped the car and looked myself over. My ribs ached pretty uniformly as though a light road roller had passed over them and there was a tender area on my left buttock where I had landed on my calipers but otherwise I seemed to have escaped damage. I removed a few spicules of wood from my trousers, got back into the car and consulted my list of visits.

And when I read my next call a gentle smile of relief spread over my face. 'Mrs Tompkin, 14, Jasmine Terrace. Clip budgie's beak.'

Thank heaven for the infinite variety of veterinary practice. After that bull I needed something small and weak and harmless and really you can't ask for much better in that line than a budgie.

Number 14 was one of a row of small mean houses built of the cheap bricks so beloved of the jerry builders after the First World War. I armed myself with a pair of clippers and stepped on to the narrow strip of pavement which separated the door from the road. A pleasant looking red-haired woman answered my knock.

'I'm Mrs Dodds from next door,' she said. 'I keep an eye on

t'old lady. She's over eighty and lives alone. I've just been out gettin' her pension for her.'

She led me into the cramped little room. 'Here y'are, love,' she said to the old woman who sat in a corner. She put the pension book and money on the mantelpiece. 'And here's Mr Herriot come to see Peter for you.'

Mrs Tompkin nodded and smiled. 'Oh that's good. Poor little feller can't hardly eat with 'is long beak and I'm worried about him. He's me only companion, you know.'

'Yes, I understand, Mrs Tompkin.' I looked at the cage by the window with the green budgie perched inside. 'These little birds can be wonderful company when they start chattering.'

She laughed. 'Aye, but it's a funny thing. Peter never has said owt much. I think he's lazy! But I just like havin' him with me.'

'Of course you do,' I said. 'But he certainly needs attention now.'

The beak was greatly overgrown, curving away down till it touched the feathers of the breast. I would be able to revolutionise his life with one quick snip from my clippers. The way I was feeling this job was right up my street.

I opened the cage door and slowly inserted my hand.

'Come on, Peter,' I wheedled as the bird fluttered away from me. And I soon cornered him and enclosed him gently in my fingers. As I lifted him out I felt in my pocket with the other hand for the clippers, but as I poised them I stopped.

The tiny head was no longer poking cheekily from my fingers but had fallen loosely to one side. The eyes were closed. I stared at the bird uncomprehendingly for a moment then opened my hand. He lay quite motionless on my palm. He was dead.

Dry mouthed, I continued to stare; at the beautiful iridescence of the plumage, the long beak which I didn't have to cut now, but mostly at the head dropping down over my forefinger. I hadn't squeezed him or been rough with him in any way but he was dead. It must have been sheer fright.

Mrs Dodds and I looked at each other in horror and I hardly dared turn my head towards Mrs Tompkin. When I did, I was surprised to see that she was still nodding and smiling.

I drew her neighbour to one side. 'Mrs Dodds, how much does she see?'

'Oh, she's very short-sighted but she's right vain despite her age. Never would wear glasses. She's hard of hearin', too.'

'Well look,' I said. My heart was still pounding. 'I just don't know what to do. If I tell her about this the shock will be terrible. Anything could happen.'

Mrs Dodds nodded, stricken-faced. 'Aye, you're right. She's that attached to the little thing.'

'I can only think of one alternative,' I whispered. 'Do you know where I can get another budgie?'

Mrs Dodds thought for a moment. 'You could try Jack Almond at t'town end. I think he keeps birds.'

I cleared my throat but even then my voice came out in a dry croak. 'Mrs Tompkin, I'm just going to take Peter along to the surgery to do this job. I won't be long.'

I left her still nodding and smiling and, cage in hand, fled into the street. I was at the town end and knocking at Jack Almond's door within three minutes.

'Mr Almond?' I asked the stout, shirtsleeved man who answered.

'That's right, young man.' He gave me a slow, placid smile. 'Do you keep birds?'

He drew himself up with dignity. 'I do, and I'm t'president of the Darrowby and Houlton Cage Bird Society.'

'Fine,' I said breathlessly. 'Have you got a green budgie?'

'Ah've got Canaries, Budgies, Parrots, Parakeets. Cockatoos ...'

'I just want a budgie.'

'Well ah've got Albinos, Blue-greens, Barreds, Litinos ...'

'I just want a green one.'

A slightly pained expression flitted across the man's face as though he found my attitude of haste somewhat unseemly.

'Aye ... well, we'll go and have a look,' he said.

I followed him as he paced unhurriedly through the house into the back yard which was largely given over to a long shed containing a bewildering variety of birds.

Mr Almond gazed at them with gentle pride and his mouth opened as though he was about to launch into a dissertation then he seemed to remember that he had an impatient chap to deal with and dragged himself back to the job in hand.

'There's a nice little green 'un here. But he's a bit older than t'others. Matter of fact I've got 'im talkin'.'

'All the better, just the thing. How much do you want for him?'

'But . . . there's some nice 'uns along here. Just let me show you . . .'

I put a hand on his arm. 'I want that one. How much?'

He pursed his lips in frustration then shrugged his shoulders. 'Ten bob.'

'Right. Bung him in this cage.'

As I sped back up the road I looked in the driving mirror and could see the poor man regarding me sadly from his doorway.

Mrs Dodds was waiting for me back at Jasmine Terrace.

'Do you think I'm doing the right thing?' I asked her in a whisper.

'I'm sure you are,' she replied. 'Poor awd thing, she hasn't much to think about and I'm sure she'd fret over Peter.'

'That's what I thought.' I made my way into the living room.

Mrs Tompkin smiled at me as I went in. 'That wasn't a long job, Mr Herriot.'

'No,' I said, hanging the cage with the new bird up in its place by the window. 'I think you'll find all is well now.'

It was months before I had the courage to put my hand into a budgie's cage again. In fact to this day I prefer it if the owners will lift the birds out for me. People look at me strangely when I ask them to do this; I believe they think I am scared the little things might bite me.

It was a long time, too, before I dared go back to Mrs Tompkin's but I was driving down Jasmine Terrace one day and on an impulse I stopped outside Number 14.

The old lady herself came to the door.

'How . . .' I said. 'How is . . . er . . . ?'

She peered at me closely for a moment then laughed. 'Oh I see who it is now. You mean Peter, don't you, Mr Herriot. Oh 'e's just grand. Come in and see 'im.'

In the little room the cage still hung by the window and Peter the Second took a quick look at me then put on a little act for my benefit; he hopped around the bars of the cage, ran up and down his ladder and rang his little bell a couple of times before returning to his perch.

His mistress reached up, tapped the metal and looked lovingly at him.

'You know, you wouldn't believe it,' she said. 'He's like a different bird.'

I swallowed. 'Is that so? In what way?'

'Well he's so active now. Lively as can be. You know 'e chatters to me all day long. It's wonderful what cuttin' a beak can do.'

6

This was one for Granville Bennett. I liked a bit of small animal surgery and was gradually doing more as time went on but this one frightened me. A twelve-year-old spaniel bitch in the last stages of pyometritis, pus dripping from her vulva on to the surgery table, temperature a hundred and four, panting, trembling, and, as I held my stethoscope against her chest I could hear the classical signs of valvular insufficiency. A dicky heart was just what I needed on top of everything else.

'Drinking a lot of water, is she?' I asked.

Old Mrs Barker twisted the strings of her shopping bag anxiously. 'Aye, she never seems to be away from the water bowl. But she won't eat – hasn't had a bite for the last four days.'

'Well I don't know,' I took off my stethoscope and stuffed it in my pocket. 'You should have brought her in long ago. She must have been ill for weeks.'

'Not rightly ill, but a bit off it. I thought there was nothing to worry about as long as she was eating.'

I didn't say anything for a few moments. I had no desire to upset the old girl but she had to be told.

'I'm afraid this is rather serious, Mrs Barker. The condition has been building up for a long time. It's in her womb, you see, a bad infection, and the only cure is an operation.'

'Well will you do it, please?' The old lady's lips quivered.

I came round the table and put my hand on her shoulder.

'I'd like to, but there are snags. She's in poor shape and twelve years old. Really a poor operation risk. I'd like to take her through to the Veterinary Hospital at Hartington and let Mr Bennett operate on her.'

'All right,' she said, nodding eagerly. 'I don't care what it costs.'

'Oh we'll keep it down as much as possible.' I walked along the passage with her and showed her out of the door. 'Leave her with me – I'll look after her, don't worry. What's her name, by the way?'

'Dinah,' she replied huskily, still peering past me down the passage.

I went through and lifted the phone. Thirty years ago country practitioners had to turn to the small animal experts when anything unusual cropped up in that line. It is different nowadays when our practices are more mixed. In Darrowby now we have the staff and equipment to tackle any type of small animal surgery but it was different then. I had heard it said that sooner or later every large animal man had to scream for help from Granville Bennett and now it was my turn.

'Hello, is that Mr Bennett?'

'It is indeed.' A big voice, friendly, full of give.

'Herriot here. I'm with Farnon in Darrowby.'

'Of course! Heard of you, laddie, heard of you.'

'Oh . . . er . . . thanks. Look, I've got a bit of a sticky job here. I wonder if you'd take it on for me?'

'Delighted, laddie, what is it?'

'A real stinking pyo.'

'Oh lovely!'

'The bitch is twelve years old.'

'Splendid!'

'And toxic as hell.'

'Excellent!'

'And one of the worst hearts I've heard for a long time.'

'Fine, fine! When are you coming through?'

'This evening, if it's OK with you. About eight.'

'Couldn't be better, laddie. See you.'

Hartington was a fair-sized town – about 200,000 inhabitants – but as I drove into the centre the traffic had thinned and only a few cars rolled past the rows of shop fronts. I hoped my twenty-five mile journey had been worth it. Dinah, stretched out on a blanket in the back looked as if she didn't care either way. I glanced behind me at the head drooping over the edge of the seat, at the white muzzle and the cataracts in her eyes gleaming palely in the light from the dash. She looked so old. Maybe I was wasting my time, placing too much faith in this man's reputation.

There was no doubt Granville Bennett had become something of a legend in northern England. In those days when specialisation was almost unknown he had gone all out for small animal work – never looked at farm stock – and had set a new standard by the modern procedures in his animal hospital which was run as nearly as possible on human lines. It was, in fact, fashionable for veterinary surgeons of that era to belittle dog and cat work; a lot of the older men who had spent their lives among the teeming thousands of draught horses in city and agriculture would sneer, 'Oh I've no time to bother with those damn things.' Bennett had gone dead in the opposite direction.

I had never met him but I knew he was a young man in his early thirties. I had heard a lot about his skill, his business acumen, and about his reputation as a *bon viveur*. He was, they

45

said, a dedicated devotee of the work-hard-play-hard school.

The Veterinary Hospital was a long low building near the top of a busy street. I drove into a yard and knocked at a door in the corner. I was looking with some awe at a gleaming Bentley dwarfing my own battered little Austin when the door was opened by a pretty receptionist.

'Good evening,' she murmured with a dazzling smile which I thought must be worth another half crown on the bill for a start. 'Do come in, Mr Bennett is expecting you.'

I was shown into a waiting room with magazines and flowers on a corner table and many impressive photographs of dogs and cats on the walls – taken, I learned later, by the principal himself. I was looking closely at a superb study of two white poodles when I heard a footstep behind me. I turned and had my first view of Granville Bennett.

He seemed to fill the room. Not over tall but of tremendous bulk. Fat, I thought at first, but as he came nearer it seemed to me that the tissue of which he was composed wasn't distributed like fat. He wasn't flabby, he didn't stick out in any particular place, he was just a big, wide, solid, hard-looking man. From the middle of a pleasant blunt-featured face the most magnificent pipe I had ever seen stuck forth shining and glorious, giving out delicious wisps of expensive smoke. It was an enormous pipe, in fact it would have looked downright silly with a smaller man, but on him it was a thing of beauty. I had a final impression of a beautifully cut dark suit and sparkling shirt cuffs as he held out a hand.

'James Herriot!' He said it as somebody else might have said 'Winston Churchill', or 'Stanley Matthews'.

'That's right.'

'Well, this is grand. Jim, is it?'

'Well yes, usually.'

'Lovely. We've got everything laid on for you, Jim. The girls are waiting in the theatre.'

'That's very kind of you, Mr Bennett.'

'Granville, Granville please!' He put his arm through mine and led me to the operating room.

Dinah was already there, looking very woebegone. She had had a sedative injection and her head nodded wearily. Bennett went over to her and gave her a swift examination.

'Mm, yes, let's get on, then.'

The two girls went into action like cogs in a smooth machine. Bennett kept a large lay staff and these animal nurses, both attractive, clearly knew what they were about. While one of them pulled up the anaesthetic and instrument trolleys the other seized Dinah's foreleg expertly above the elbow, raised the radial vein by pressure and quickly clipped and disinfected the area.

The big man strolled up with a loaded needle and effortlessly slipped the needle into the vein.

'Pentothal,' he said as Dinah slowly collapsed and lay unconscious on the table. It was one of the new short-acting anaesthetics which I had never seen used.

While Bennett scrubbed up and donned sterilised gown and cap the girls rolled Dinah on her back and secured her there with ties to loops on the operating table. They applied the ether and oxygen mask to her face then shaved and swabbed the operation site. The big man returned in time to have a scalpel placed in his hand.

With almost casual speed he incised skin and muscle layers and when he went through the peritoneum the horns of the uterus which in normal health would have been two slim pink ribbons now welled into the wound like twin balloons, swollen and turgid with pus. No wonder Dinah had felt ill, carrying that lot around with her.

The stubby fingers tenderly worked round the mass, ligated the ovarian vessels and uterine body then removed the whole thing and dropped it into an enamel bowl. It wasn't till he had begun to stitch that I realised that the operation was nearly over though he had been at the table for only a few minutes. It would all have looked childishly easy except that his total involvement showed in occasional explosive commands to the nurses.

And as I watched him working under the shadowless lamp with the white tiled walls around him and the rows of instruments gleaming by his side it came to me with a rush of mixed emotions that this was what I had always wanted to do myself. My dreams when I had first decided on veterinary work had been precisely of this. Yet here I was, a somewhat shaggy cow doctor; or perhaps more correctly a farm physician, but certainly something very different. The scene before me was a far cry from my routine of kicks and buffets, of muck and sweat. And yet I had no regrets; the life which had been forced on me by circumstances had turned out to be a thing of magical fulfilment. It came to me with a flooding certainty that I would rather spend my days driving over the unfenced roads of the high country than stooping over that operating table.

And anyway I couldn't have been a Bennett. I don't think I could have matched his technique and this whole set up was eloquent of a lot of things like business sense, foresight and driving ambition which I just didn't possess.

My colleague was finished now and was fitting up an intravenous saline drip. He taped the needle down in the vein then turned to me.

'That's it, then, Jim. It's up to the old girl now.' He began to lead me from the room and it struck me how very pleasant it must be to finish your job and walk away from it like this. In Darrowby I'd have been starting now to wash the instruments, scrub the table, and the final scene would have been of Herriot the great surgeon swilling the floor with mop and bucket. This was a better way.

Back in the waiting room Bennett pulled on his jacket and extracted from a side pocket the immense pipe which he inspected with a touch of anxiety as if he feared mice had been nibbling at it in his absence. He wasn't satisfied with his examination because he brought forth a soft yellow cloth and began to polish the briar with intense absorption. Then he held the pipe high, moving it slightly from side to side, his eyes softening at the play of the light on the exquisite grain. Finally he produced a pouch of mammoth proportions, filled the bowl, applied a match with a touch of reverence and closed his eyes as a fragrant mist drifted from his lips.

'That baccy smells marvellous,' I said. 'What is it?'

'Navy Cut De Luxe.' He closed his eyes again. 'You know, I could eat the smoke.'

I laughed. 'I use the ordinary Navy Cut myself.'

He gazed at me like a sorrowing Buddha, 'Oh you mustn't, laddie, you mustn't. This is the only stuff. Rich . . . fruity . . .' His hand made languid motions in the air. 'Here, you can take some away with you.'

He pulled open a drawer. I had a brief view of a stock which wouldn't have disgraced a fair-sized tobacconist's shop; innumerable tins, pipes, cleaners, reamers, cloths.

'Try this,' he said, 'and tell me if I'm not right.'

I looked down at the first container in my hand. 'Oh but I can't take all this. It's a four ounce tin!'

'Rubbish, my boy. Put it in your pocket.' He became suddenly brisk. 'Now I expect you'll want to hang around till old Dinah comes out of the anaesthetic so why don't we have a quick beer? I'm a member of a nice little club just across the road.'

'Well fine, sounds great.'

He moved lightly and swiftly for a big man and I had to hurry to keep up with him as he left the surgery and crossed to a building on the other side of the street.

7

Inside the club was masculine comfort, hails of welcome from some prosperous looking members and a friendly greeting from the man behind the bar.

'Two pints, Fred,' murmured Bennett absently, and the drinks appeared with amazing speed. My colleague poured his down apparently without swallowing and turned to me.

'Another, Jim?'

I had just tried a sip at mine and began to gulp anxiously at the bitter ale. 'Right, but let me get this one.'

'No can do, laddie.' He glanced at me with mild severity. 'Only members can buy drinks. Same again, Fred.'

I found I had two glasses at my elbow and with a tremendous effort I got the first one down. Gasping slightly I was surveying the second one timidly when I noticed that Bennett was three-quarters down his. As I watched he drained it effortlessly.

'You're slow, Jim,' he said, smiling indulgently. 'Just set them up again will you, Fred.'

In some alarm I watched the barman ply his handle and attacked my second pint resolutely. I surprised myself by forcing it over my tonsils then, breathing heavily, I got hold of the third one just as Bennett spoke again.

'We'll just have one for the road, Jim,' he said pleasantly. 'Would you be so kind, Fred?'

This was ridiculous but I didn't want to appear a piker at our first meeting. With something akin to desperation I raised the third and began to suck feebly at it. When my glass was empty I almost collapsed against the counter. My stomach was agonisingly distended and a light perspiration had broken out on my brow. As I almost lay there I saw my colleague moving across the carpet towards the door.

'Time we were off, Jim,' he said. 'Drink up.'

It's wonderful what the human frame can tolerate when put to the test. I would have taken bets that it was impossible for me to drink that fourth pint without at least half an hour's rest, preferably in the prone position, but as Bennett's shoe tapped impatiently I tipped the beer a little at a time into my mouth, feeling it wash around my back teeth before incredibly disappearing down my gullet. I believe the water torture was a favourite with the Spanish Inquisition and as the pressure inside me increased I knew just how their victims felt.

When I at last blindly replaced my glass and splashed my way from the bar the big man was holding the door open. Outside in the street he placed an arm across my shoulder.

'The old Spaniel won't be out of it yet,' he said. 'We'll just slip to my house and have a bite – I'm a little peckish.'

Sunk in the deep upholstery of the Bentley, cradling my swollen abdomen in my arms I watched the shop fronts flicker past the windows and give way to the darkness of the open countryside. We drew up outside a fine grey stone house in a typical Yorkshire village and Bennett ushered me inside.

He pushed me towards a leather armchair. 'Make yourself at home, laddie. Zoe's out at the moment but I'll get some grub.' He bustled through to the kitchen and reappeared in seconds with a deep bowl which he placed on a table by my side.

'You know, Jim,' he said, rubbing his hands. 'There's nothing better after beer than a few pickled onions.'

I cast a timorous glance into the bowl. Everything in this man's life seemed to be larger than life, even the onions. They were bigger than golf balls, brownish-white, glistening.

'Well thanks Mr Ben . . . Granville.' I took one of them, held it between finger and thumb and stared at it helplessly. The beer hadn't even begun to sort itself out inside me; the idea of starting on this potent-looking vegetable was unthinkable.

Granville reached into the bowl, popped an onion into his mouth, crunched it quickly, swallowed and sank his teeth into a second. 'By God, that's good. You know, my little wife's a marvellous cook. She even makes pickled onions better than anyone.'

Munching happily he moved over to the sideboard and clinked around for a few moments before placing in my hand a heavy cut glass tumbler about two thirds full of neat whisky. I couldn't say anything because I had taken the plunge and put the onion in my mouth; and as I bit boldly into it the fumes rolled in a volatile wave into my nasal passages, making me splutter. I took a gulp at the whisky and looked up at Granville with watering eyes.

He was holding out the onion bowl again and when I declined he regarded it for a moment with hurt in his eyes. 'It's funny you don't like them, I always thought Zoe did them marvellously.'

'Oh you're wrong, Granville, they're delicious. I just haven't finished this one.'

He didn't reply but continued to look at the bowl with gentle sorrow. I realised there was nothing else for it; I took another onion.

Immensely gratified, Granville hurried through to the kitchen again. This time when he came back he bore a tray with an enormous cold roast, a loaf of bread, butter and mustard.

'I think a beef sandwich would go down rather nicely, Jim,' he murmured, as he stropped his carving knife on a steel. Then he noticed my glass of whisky still half full.

'C'mon, c'mon, c'mon!' he said with some asperity. 'You're not touching your drink.' He watched me benevolently as I drained the glass then he refilled it to its old level. 'That's better. And have another onion.'

I stretched my legs out and rested my head on the back of the chair in an attempt to ease my internal turmoil. My stomach was a lake of volcanic lava bubbling and popping fiercely in its crater with each additional piece of onion, every sip of whisky setting up a fresh violent reaction. Watching Granville at work, a great wave of nausea swept over me. He was sawing busily at the roast, carving off slices which looked to be an inch thick, slapping mustard on them and enclosing them in the bread. He hummed with contentment as the pile grew. Every now and then he had another onion.

'Now then, laddie,' he cried at length, putting a heaped plate at my elbow. 'Get yourself round that lot.' He took his own supply and collapsed with a sigh into another chair.

He took a gargantuan bite and spoke as he chewed. 'You know, Jim, this is something I enjoy – a nice little snack. Zoe always leaves me plenty to go at when she pops out.' He engulfed a further few inches of sandwich. 'And I'll tell you something, though I say it myself, these are bloody good, don't you think so?'

'Yes indeed.' Squaring my shoulders I bit, swallowed and held my breath as another unwanted foreign body slid down to the ferment below.

Just then I heard the front door open.

'Ah, that'll be Zoe,' Granville said, and was about to rise when a disgracefully fat Staffordshire Bull Terrier burst into the room, waddled across the carpet and leapt into his lap.

'Phoebles, my dear, come to daddykins!' he shouted. 'Have you had nice walkies with mummy?'

The Staffordshire was closely followed by a Yorkshire Terrier which was also enthusiastically greeted by Granville.

'Yoo-hoo, Victoria, yoo-hoo!'

The Yorkie, an obvious smiler, did not jump up but contented herself with sitting at her master's feet, baring her teeth ingratiatingly every few seconds.

I smiled through my pain. Another myth exploded; the one about these specialist small animal vets not being fond of dogs themselves. The big man crooned over the two little animals. The fact that he called Phoebe 'Phoebles' was symptomatic.

I heard light footsteps in the hall and looked up expectantly. I had Granville's wife taped neatly in my mind; domesticated, devoted, homely; many of these dynamic types had wives like that, willing slaves content to lurk in the background. I waited confidently for the entrance of a plain little hausfrau.

When the door opened I almost let my vast sandwich fall. Zoe Bennett was a glowing warm beauty who would make any man alive stop for another look. A lot of soft brown hair, large grey-green friendly eyes, a tweed suit sitting sweetly on a slim but not too slim figure; and something else, a wholesomeness, an inner light which made me wish suddenly that I was a better man or at least that I looked better than I did.

In an instant I was acutely conscious of the fact that my shoes were dirty, that my old jacket and corduroy trousers were out of place here. I hadn't troubled to change but had rushed straight out in my working clothes, and they were different from Granville's because I couldn't go round the farms in a suit like his.

'My love, my love!' he carolled joyously as his wife bent over and kissed him fondly. 'Let me introduce Jim Herriot from Darrowby.'

The beautiful eyes turned on me.

'How d'you do, Mr Herroit!' She looked as pleased to see me as her husband had done and again I had the desperate wish that I was more presentable; that my hair was combed, that I didn't have this mounting conviction that I was going to explode into a thousand pieces at any moment.

'I'm going to have a cup of tea, Mr Herroit. Would you like one?'

'No-no, no no, thank you very much but no, no, not at the moment.' I backed away slightly.

'Ah well, I see you've got one of Granville's little sandwiches.' She giggled and went to get her tea.

When she came back she handed a parcel to her husband. 'I've been shopping today, darling. Picked up some of those shirts you like so much.'

'My sweet! How kind of you!' He began to tear at the brown paper like a schoolboy and produced three elegant shirts in cellophane covers. 'They're marvellous, my pet, you spoil me.' He looked up at me. 'Jim! These are the most wonderful shirts, you must have one.' He flicked a shining package across the room on to my lap.

I looked down at it in amazement. 'No, really I can't . . .'

'Of course you can. You keep it.'

'But Granville, not a shirt . . . it's too . . .'

'It's a very good shirt.' He was beginning to look hurt again. I subsided.

They were both so kind. Zoe sat right by me with her tea cup, chatting pleasantly, while Granville beamed at me from his chair as he finished the last of the sandwiches and started again on the onions.

The proximity of the attractive woman was agreeable but embarrassing. My corduroys in the warmth of the room had begun to give off the unmistakable bouquet of the farmyard where they spent most of their time. And though it was one of my favourite scents there was no doubt it didn't go with these elegant surroundings.

And worse still, I had started a series of internal rumblings and musical tinklings which resounded only too audibly during

54

every lull in the conversation. The only other time I have heard such sounds was in a cow with an advanced case of displacement of the abomasum. My companions delicately feigned deafness even when I produced a shameful, explosive belch which made the little fat dog start up in alarm, but when another of these mighty borborygmi escaped me and almost made the windows rattle I thought it time to go.

In any case I wasn't contributing much else. The alcohol had taken hold and I was increasingly conscious that I was just sitting there with a stupid leer on my face. In striking contrast to Granville who looked just the same as when I first met him back at the surgery. He was cool and possessed, his massive urbanity unimpaired. It was a little hard.

So, with the tin of tobacco bumping against my hip and the shirt tucked under my arm I took my leave.

Back at the hospital I looked down at Dinah. The old dog had come through wonderfully well and she lifted her head and gazed at me sleepily. Her colour was good and her pulse strong. The operative shock had been dramatically minimised by my colleague's skilful speedy technique and by the intravenous drip.

I knelt down and stroked her ears. 'You know, I'm sure she's going to make it, Granville.'

Above me the great pipe nodded with majestic confidence.

'Of course, laddie, of course.'

And he was right. Dinah was rejuvenated by her hysterectomy and lived to delight her mistress for many more years.

On the way home that night she lay by my side on the passenger seat, her nose poking from a blanket. Now and then she rested her chin on my hand as it gripped the gear lever and occasionally she licked me lazily.

I could see she felt better than I did.

8

As I looked at the group of sick young cattle on the hillside a mixture of apprehension and disbelief flooded through me. Surely not more trouble for the Dalbys.

The old saw 'It never rains but it pours' seems to apply with particular force to farming. The husk outbreak last year and now this. It had all started with the death of Billy Dalby; big, slow-smiling, slow-talking Billy. He was as strong and tough as any of the shaggy beasts which ranged his fields but he had just melted away in a few weeks. Cancer of the pancreas they said it was and Billy was gone before anybody could realise it and there was only his picture smiling down from the kitchen mantelpiece on his wife and three young children.

The general opinion was that Mrs Dalby should sell up and get out. You needed a man to run this place and anyway Prospect House was a bad farm. Neighbouring farmers would stick out their lower lips and shake their heads when they looked at the boggy pastures on the low side of the house with the tufts of spiky grass sticking from the sour soil or at the rocky outcrops and scattered stones on the hillside fields. No, it was a poor place and a woman would never make a go of it.

Everybody thought the same thing except Mrs Dalby herself. There wasn't much of her, in fact she must have been one of the smallest women I have ever seen – around five feet high – but there was a core of steel in her. She had her own mind and her own way of doing things.

I remember when Billy was still alive I had been injecting some sheep up there and Mrs Dalby called me into the house.

'You'll have a cup of tea, Mr Herriot?' She said it in a gracious way, not casually, her head slightly on one side and a dignified little smile on her face.

And when I went into the kitchen I knew what I would find; the inevitable tray. It was always a tray with Mrs Dalby. The hospitable Dales people were continually asking me in for some kind of refreshment – a 'bit o' dinner' perhaps, but if it wasn't midday there was usually a mug of tea and a scone or a hunk of thick-crusted apple pie – but Mrs Dalby invariably set out a special tray. And there it was today with a clean cloth and the best china cup and saucer and side plates with sliced buttered scones and iced cakes and malt bread and biscuits. It was on its own table away from the big kitchen table.

'Do sit down, Mr Herriot,' she said in her precise manner. 'I hope that tea isn't too strong for you.'

Her speech was what the farmers would call 'very proper' but it went with her personality which to me embodied a determination to do everything as correctly as possible.

'Looks perfect to me, Mrs Dalby.' I sat down, feeling somewhat exposed, in the middle of the kitchen with Billy smiling comfortably from an old armchair by the fire and his wife standing by my side.

She never sat down with us but stood there, very erect, hands clasped in front of her, head inclined, ceremoniously attending to my every wish. 'Let me fill your cup, Mr Herriot,' or 'Won't you try some of this custard tart?'

She wasn't what you would call pretty; it was a rough-skinned red little face with tiny, very dark eyes but there was a sweet expression and a quiet dignity. And as I say, there was strength.

Billy died in the spring and as everybody waited for Mrs Dalby to make arrangement for the sale she went right on with the running of the farm. She did it with the help of a big farm worker called Charlie who had helped Billy occasionally but now came full time. During the summer I was called out a few times for trivial ailments among the cattle and I could see that Mrs Dalby was managing to hang on; she looked a bit haggard because she was now helping in the fields and buildings as well as coping with her housework and young family, but she was still fighting.

It was half way through September when she asked me to call to see some young cattle – stirks of around nine months – which were coughing.

'They were really fit when they were turned out in May,' she said, as we walked across the grass to the gate in the corner. 'But they've gone down badly this last week or two.'

I held the gate open, we walked through, and as I approached the group of animals I grew progressively uneasy. Even at this distance I could see that something was far wrong; they were not moving around or grazing as they should have been but were curiously immobile. There would be about thirty of them and many had their necks extended forward as if seeking air. And from the bunch a barking cough was carried to us on the soft breeze of late summer.

By the time we reached the cattle my uneasiness had been replaced by a dry-mouthed dread. They didn't seem to care as I moved in among them and I had to shout and wave my arms to get them moving; and they had barely begun to stir before the coughing broke out throughout the group; not just an occasional bark but a hacking chorus which seemed almost to be tearing the little animals apart. And they weren't just coughing; most of them were panting, standing straddle-legged, ribs heaving in a desperate fight for breath. A few showed bubbles of saliva at their lips and from here and there among the pack groans of agony sounded as the lungs laboured.

I turned as in a dream to Mrs Dalby.

'They've got husk.' Even as I said it it sounded a grimly inadequate description of the tragedy I was witnessing. Because this was neglected husk, a terrible doom-laden thing.

'Husk?' the little woman said brightly. 'What causes it?'

I looked at her for a moment then tried to make my voice casual.

'Well it's a parasite. A tiny worm which infests the bronchial tubes and sets up bronchitis – in fact that's the proper name, parasitic bronchitis. The larvae climb up the blades of grass and the cattle eat them as they graze. Some pastures are badly affected with it.' I broke off. A lecture was out of place at a time like this.

What I felt like saying was why in God's name hadn't I been called in weeks ago. Because this wasn't only bronchitis now; it was pneumonia, pleurisy, emphysema and any other lung

58

condition you cared to name with not merely a few of the hair-like worms irritating the tubes, but great seething masses of them crawling everywhere, balling up and blocking the vital air passages. I had opened up a lot of calves like these and I knew how it looked.

I took a deep breath. 'They're pretty bad, Mrs Dalby. A mild attack isn't so bad if you can get them off the grass right away, but this has gone a long way beyond that. You can see for your-self, can't you – they're like a lot of little skeletons. I wish I'd seen them sooner.'

She looked up at me apprehensively and I decided not to belabour the point. It would be like rubbing it in; saying what her neighbours had said all along, that her inexperience would land her in trouble sooner or later. If Billy had been here he probably would never have turned his young cattle on to this marshy field; or he would have spotted the trouble right at the start and brought them inside. Charlie would be no help in a situation like this; he was a good willing chap but lived up to the Yorkshire saying, 'Strong in t'arm and thick in t'head.' Farming is a skilful business and Billy, the planner, the stocks-man, the experienced agriculturist who knew his own farm in-side out, just wasn't there.

Mrs Dalby drew herself up with that familiar gesture.

'Well what can we do about it, Mr Herriot?'

An honest reply in those days would have been, 'Medicinally nothing.' But I didn't say that.

'We've got to get them all inside immediately. Every mouth-ful of this grass is adding to the worm burden. Is Charlie around to give us a hand?'

'Yes, he's in the next field, mending a wall.' She trotted across the turf and in a minute or two returned with the big man ambling by her side.

'Aye, ah thought it were a touch of husk,' he said amiably, then with a hint of eagerness, 'Are ye goin' to give them the throat injection?'

'Yes . . . yes . . . but let's get them up to the buildings.' As we drove the cattle slowly up the green slope I marvelled ruefully at this further example of faith in the intratracheal injection for husk. There was really no treatment for the condition and it would be another twenty years before one appeared in the shape of diethylcarbamazine, but the accepted procedure was to inject a mixture of chloroform, turpentine and creosote into the windpipe. Modern vets may raise their eyebrows at the idea of introducing this barbaric concoction directly into the delicate lung tissue and we old ones didn't think much of it either. But the farmers loved it.

When we had finally got the stirks into the fold yard I looked round with something like despair. The short journey had exacerbated their symptoms tremendously and I stood in the middle of a symphony of coughs, grunts and groans while the cattle, tongues protruding, ribs pumping, gasped for breath.

I got a bottle of the wonderful injection from the car, and with Charlie holding the head and little Mrs Dalby hanging on to the tail I began to go through the motions. Seizing the trachea in my left hand I inserted the needle between the cartilaginous rings and squirted a few c.c.'s into the lumen and, as always, the stirk gave a reflex cough, sending up the distinctive aroma of the medicaments into our faces.

'By gaw, you can smell it straight off, guvnor,' Charlie said with deep satisfaction. 'Ye can tell it's gettin' right to t'spot.'

Most of the farmers said something like that. And they had faith. The books spoke comfortably about the chloroform stupefying the worms, the turpentine killing them and the creosote causing increased coughing which expelled them. But I didn't believe a word of it. The good results which followed were in my opinion due entirely to bringing the animals in from the infected pasture.

But I knew I had to do it and we injected every animal in the yard. There were thirty-two of them and Mrs Dalby's tiny figure was involved in the catching of all of them; clutching vainly at their necks, grabbing their tails, pushing them up against the wall. William, the eldest son, aged eight, came in from school and plunged into the fray by his mother's side.

My repeated 'Be careful, Mrs Dalby!' or Charlie's gruff

'Watch thissen, Missis, or you'll get lamed!' had no effect. During the mêlée both she and the little boy were kicked, trodden on and knocked down but they never showed the slightest sign of being discouraged.

At the end, the little woman turned to me, her face flushed to an even deeper hue. Panting, she looked up. 'Is there anything else we can do, Mr Herriot?'

'Yes there is.' In fact the two things I was going to tell her were the only things which ever did any good. 'First, I'm going to leave you some medicine for the worms which are in the stomach. We can get at them there, so Charlie must give every stirk a dose. Secondly, you'll have to start giving them the best possible food – good hay and high protein cake.'

Her eyes widened. 'Cake? That's expensive stuff. And hay...'

I knew what she was thinking. The precious hay safely garnered for next winter's feed; to have to start using it now was a cruel blow, especially with all that beautiful grass out there; grass, the most natural, most perfect food for cattle but every blade carrying its own load of death.

'Can't they go out again ... ever?' she asked in a small voice.

'No, I'm sorry. If they had just had a mild attack you could have kept them in at nights and turned them out after the dew had left the grass in the mornings. The larvae climb up the grass mainly when it's wet. But your cattle have got too far. We daren't risk them picking up any more worms.'

'Right ... thank you, Mr Herriot. We know where we are, anyway.' She paused. 'Do you think we'll lose any of them?'

My stomach contracted into a tight ball. I had already told her to buy cake she couldn't afford and it was a certainty she would have to lay out more precious cash for hay in the winter. How was I going to tell her that nothing in the world was going to stop this batch of beasts dying like flies? When animals with husk started blowing bubbles it was nearly hopeless and the ones which were groaning with every breath were quite simply doomed. Nearly half of them were in these two categories and what about the rest? The pathetic barking other half? Well, they had a chance.

'Mrs Dalby,' I said, 'it would be wrong of me to make light of this. Some of them are going to die, in fact unless there's a miracle you are going to lose quite a few of them.' At the sight of her stricken face I made an attempt to be encouraging. 'However, where there's life there's hope and sometimes you get pleasant surprises at this job.' I held up a finger. 'Worm them and get some good grub into them! That's your hope – to help them fight it off themselves.'

'I see.' She lifted her chin in her characteristic way. 'And now you must come in for a wash.'

And of course there it was in its usual place in the kitchen; the tray with all the trimmings.

'Really, Mrs Dalby. You shouldn't have bothered. You have enough to do without this.'

'Nonsense,' she said, the smile back on her face. 'You take one spoonful of sugar don't you?'

As I sat there she stood in her habitual position, hands clasped in front of her, watching me while the middle boy, Dennis, who was five, looked up at me solemnly and Michael, a mere toddler of two, fell over the coal scuttle and started to bawl lustily.

The usual procedure was to repeat the intratracheal injection in four days so I had to go through with it. Anyway, it gave me a chance to see how the cattle were faring.

When I drew up in the yard my first sight was of a long sack-covered mound on the cobbles. A row of hooves protruded from beneath the sacks. I had expected something of the sort but the reality was still like a blow in the face. It was still quite early in the morning and perhaps I wasn't feeling quite strong enough to have the evidence of my failure thrust before my eyes. Because failure it undoubtedly was; even though I had been in a hopeless position from the start there was something damning in those motionless hooves jutting from their rough blanket.

I made a quick count. There were four dead cattle under there. Wearily I made my way into the fold yard; I had no cheerful expectation of what I would find inside. Two of the stirks were down and unable to rise from the deep straw, the rest were still panting, but I noticed with a faint lifting of my gloom that several of them were doggedly munching at the cubes of cake in the troughs and other were pulling an occasional wisp of hay from the racks. It was incredible how animals with advanced respiratory symptoms would still eat; and it provided the only gleam of hope.

I walked over to the house. Mrs Dalby greeted me cheerfully as though those carcases outside didn't exist.

'It's time for the second injection,' I said, and then after some hesitation, 'I see you've lost four of them . . . I'm sorry.'

'Well you told me, Mr Herriot.' She smiled through the tired lines on her face. 'You said I had to expect it so it wasn't as big a shock as it might have been.' She finished washing the youngest child's face, seized a towel in her work-roughened hands and rubbed him briskly, then she straightened up. It was Saturday and William was at home and I noticed not for the first time that there was something about the little boy which suggested that even at his age he had decided he was going to be the man about the house. He pulled on his little wellingtons and marched resolutely with us across the yard to do his bit as he saw it. I rested my hand on his shoulder as he walked beside me; he would have to grow up a lot more rapidly than most youngsters but I had the feeling that the realities of life wouldn't bowl him over very easily.

We gave the animals their second injection with the two little Dalbys again throwing themselves fearlessly into the rough and tumble and that was about the last practical thing I did in the husk outbreak.

Looking back, there is a macabre fascination in recalling situations like this when we veterinary surgeons were utterly helpless in the face of inevitable diaster. Nowadays, thank heavens, the young members of the profession do not have to stand among a group of gasping, groaning creatures with the sick knowledge that they can't do a thing about it; they have an excellent oral vaccine to prevent husk and efficient therapeutic agents to treat it.

But with the Dalbys who needed my help so desperately I had nothing to offer; my memories are of repeated comfortless visits, of death, and of an all-pervading reek of chloroform, creosote and turpentine. When the business had finally come to an end a dozen of the stirks had died, about five were alive but blowing hard and would probably be stunted and unthrifty for the rest of their lives. The rest, thanks to the good feeding and not to my treatment, had recovered.

It was a crushing blow for any farmer to take but for a widow struggling to survive it could have been fatal. But on my last visit little Mrs Dalby, hovering as usual, hands clasped, above the tea tray, was undefeated.

'Only them as has them can lose them,' she said firmly, her head tilted as always.

I had heard that said many times and they were brave Yorkshire words. But I wondered . . . did she have enough to be able to lose so many?

She went on, 'I know you've told me not to turn the young beasts on to that field next year but isn't there anything we can give them to stop them getting husk?'

'No, Mrs Dalby, I'm sorry.' I put down my cup. 'I don't think there's anything country vets need and want more than a husk vaccine. People keep asking us that question and we have to keep on saying no.'

We had to keep on saying no for another twenty years as we watched disasters like I had just seen at the Dalbys', and the strange thing is that now we have a first rate vaccine it is taken completely for granted.

Driving away I stopped to open the gate at the end of the track and looked back at the old stone farmhouse crouching against the lower slopes. It was a perfect autumn day with mellow golden sunshine softening the harsh sweep of fell and moor with their striding walls and the air so still and windless that the whirring of a pigeon's wings overhead was loud in the silence. Across the valley on the hilltop a frieze of sparse trees stood as motionless as though they had been painted across the blue canvas of sky.

It seemed wrong that in the midst of this beauty was worry and anxiety, grinding struggle and the threat of ruin. I closed the gate and got back into the car. That little woman over there may have weathered this calamity but as I started the engine the thought was strong in my mind that another such thing would finish her.

9

I was vastly relieved when winter came and spring followed and I saw virtually nothing of Mrs Dalby. It was one market day in mid-summer that she came to the surgery. I was just going to open the door when Siegfried beat me to it. More than most people he appreciated the hospitality we were shown on the farms and he had sampled Mrs Dalby's tray as often as I had. On top of that he had the deepest admiration for her indomitable battle to keep the farm going for her children, so that whenever she appeared at Skeldale House he received her like royalty. His manners, always impeccable, became those of a Spanish grandee.

I watched him now as he threw the door wide and hurried to the top step.

'Why, Mrs Dalby! How very nice to see you! Do come inside.' He extended his hand towards the house.

The little woman, dignified as ever, inclined her head, smiled and walked past him while Siegfried hastened to her side; and as they negotiated the passage he kept up a running fire of enquiries. 'And how is William . . . and Dennis . . . and little Michael? Good, good, splendid.'

At the sitting-room door there was the same ceremonious opening and courteous gestures and once inside a tremendous scraping of armchairs as he hauled them around to make sure she was comfortable and in the right position.

65

Next he galloped through to the kitchen to organise some refreshment and when Mrs Hall appeared with the tray he raked it with an anxious glance as though he feared it might fall below the standard of Mrs Dalby's. Apparently reassured, he poured the tea, hovered around solicitously for a moment or two then sat down opposite, the very picture of rapt attention.

The little woman thanked him and sipped at her cup.

'Mr Farnon, I have called to see you about some young beasts. I turned a batch of thirty-five out this spring and they looked in good condition but now they're losing ground fast – all of them.'

My heart gave a great thump and something must have shown in my face because she smiled across at me.

'Oh don't worry, Mr Herriot, it's not husk again. There's not a cough among the lot of them. But they are going thin and they're badly scoured.'

'I think I know what that will be,' Siegfried said, leaning across to push a plate of Mrs Hall's flapjack towards her. 'They'll have picked up a few worms. Not lungworms but the stomach and intestinal kind. They probably just need a good dose of medicine to clear them out.'

She nodded and took a piece of the flapjack. 'Yes, that's what Charlie thought and we've dosed the lot of them. But it doesn't seem to have made any difference.'

'That's funny.' Siegfried rubbed his chin. 'Mind you they sometimes need a repeat but you should have seen some improvement. Perhaps we'd better have a look at them.'

'That's what I would like,' she said. 'It would set my mind at rest.'

Siegfried opened the appointment book. 'Right, and the sooner the better. Tomorrow morning all right ? Splendid.' He made a quick note then looked up at her. 'By the way I'm going off for a week's holiday starting this evening so Mr Herriot will be coming.'

'That will be fine,' she replied, turning to me and smiling without a trace of doubt or misgiving. If she was thinking 'This is the fellow who supervised the deaths of nearly half of my young stock last year' she certainly didn't show it. In fact when she finally finished her tea and left she waved and smiled again as though she could hardly wait to see me again.

And when I walked across the fields with Mrs Dalby next day it was like turning the clock back to last year, except that we were going in the other direction; not down towards the marshy ground below the house but up to the stony pastures which climbed in an uneven checkerboard between their stone walls over the lower slopes of the hill.

The similarity persisted as we approached, too. These young beasts – roans, reds, red and whites – were an almost exact counterpart of last year's batch; shaggy little creatures, little more than calves, they stood spindly-legged and knock-kneed regarding us apathetically as we came up the rise. And though their symptoms were entirely different from the previous lot there was one thing I could say for sure; they were very ill.

As I watched I could see the dark watery diarrhoea flowing from them without any lifting of the tails as though there was nothing they could do to control it. And every one of them was painfully thin, the skin stretched over the jutting pelvic bones and the protruding rows of ribs.

'I haven't neglected them this time,' Mrs Dalby said.

'I know they look dreadful but this seems to have happened within a few days.'

'Yes . . . yes . . . I see . . .' My eyes were hunting desperately among the little animals trying to find some sort of clue. I had seen unthriftiness from parasitism but nothing like this.

'Have you kept a lot of cattle in these fields over the last year or two?' I asked.

She paused in thought for a moment. 'No . . . no . . . I don't think so. Billy used to let the milk cows graze up here now and then but that's all.'

The grass wouldn't be likely to be 'sick' with worms, then. In any case it didn't look like that. What it did look like was Johne's disease, but how in God's name could thirty-five young things like this get Johne's at the same time? Salmonella . . . ? Coccidiosis . . . ? Some form of poisoning, perhaps . . . this was the time of year when cattle ate strange plants. I walked slowly round the field, but there was nothing unusual to be seen; it took even the grass all its time to grow on these wind-blown hillsides and there was no great range of other herbage. I could see bracken higher up the fell but none down here; Billy would have cleared it years ago.

'Mrs Dalby,' I said. 'I think you'd better give these stirks another dose of the worm medicine just to be sure and in the meantime I'm going to take some samples of the manure for examination at the laboratory.'

I brought up some sterile jars from the car and went painstakingly round the pasture scooping up as wide a range as possible from the pools of faeces.

I took them to the lab myself and asked them to phone the results through. The call came within twenty-four hours; negative for everything. I resisted the impulse to dash out to the farm immediately; there was nothing I could think of doing and it wouldn't look so good for me to stand there gawping at the beasts and scratching my head. Better to wait till tomorrow to see if the second dose of worm medicine did any good. There was no reason why it should, because none of the samples showed a pathogenic worm burden.

In these cases I always hope that inspiration will come to me as I am driving around or even when I am examining other animals but this time as I climbed from the car outside Prospect House I was barren of ideas.

The young beasts were slightly worse. I had decided that if I still couldn't think of anything I would give the worst ones vitamin injections more or less for the sake of doing something; so with Charlie holding the heads I inserted the hypodermic under the taut skins of ten of the little creatures, trying at the same time to put away the feeling of utter futility. We didn't have to drive them inside; they were easily caught in the open field and that was a bad sign in itself.

'Well you'll let me know, Mrs Dalby,' I said hoarsely as I got back into the car. 'If that injection improves them I'll do the lot.' I gave what I hoped was a confident wave and drove off.

I felt so bad that it had a numbing effect on me and over the next few days my mind seemed to shy away from the subject of the Dalby stirks as though by not thinking about them they would just go away. I was reminded that they were still very much there by a phone call from Mrs Dalby.

'I'm afraid my cattle aren't doing any good, Mr Herriot.' Her voice was strained.

I grimaced into the receiver. 'And the ones I injected . . . ?'

'Just the same as the others.'

I had to face up to reality now and drove out to Prospect House immediately; but the feeling of cold emptiness, of having nothing to offer, made the journey a misery. I hadn't the courage to go to the farmhouse and face Mrs Dalby but hurried straight up through the fields to where the young beasts were gathered.

And when I walked among them and studied them at close range the apprehension I had felt on the journey was nothing to the sick horror which rushed through me now. Another catastrophe was imminent here. The big follow-up blow which was all that was needed to knock the Dalby family out once and for all was on its way. These animals were going to die. Not just half of them like last year but all of them, because there was hardly any variation in their symptoms; there didn't seem to be a single one of them which was fighting off the disease.

But what disease? God almighty, I was a veterinary surgeon! Maybe not steeped in experience but I wasn't a new beginner any more. I should surely have some small inkling why a whole great batch of young beasts was sinking towards the knacker yard in front of my eyes.

I could see Mrs Dalby coming up the field with little William, striding in his tough, arm-swinging way by her side, and Charlie following behind.

What the hell was I going to say to them? Shrug my shoulders with a light laugh and say I hadn't a single clue in my head and that it would probably be best to phone Mallock now and ask them to shoot the lot of them straight away for dog meat? They wouldn't have any cattle to bring on for next year but that wouldn't matter because they would no longer be farming.

Stumbling among the stricken creatures I gazed at them in turn, almost choking as I looked at the drooping, sunken-eyed heads, the gaunt little bodies, the eternal trickle of that deadly scour. There was a curious immobility about the group, probably because they were too weak to walk about; in fact as I watched, one of them took a few steps, swayed and almost fell.

Charlie was pushing open the gate into the field just a hundred yards away. I turned and stared at the nearest animal, almost beseeching it to tell me what was wrong with it, where it felt the pain, how this thing had all started. But I got no response. The stirk, one of the smallest, only calf-size, with a very dark roan-coloured head showed not the slightest interest but gazed back at me incuriously through its spectacles. What was that . . . what was I thinking about . . . spectacles? Was my reason toppling . . . ? But yes, by God, he did have spectacles . . . a ring of lighter hair surrounding each eye. And that other beast over there . . . he was the same. Oh glory be, now I knew! At last I knew!

Mrs Dalby, panting slightly, had reached me.

'Good morning, Mr Herriot,' she said, trying to smile. 'What do you think, then?' She looked around the cattle with anxious eyes.

'Ah, good morning to you, Mrs Dalby,' I replied expansively, fighting down the impulse to leap in the air and laugh and shout and perhaps do a few cartwheels. 'Yes, I've had a look at them and it is pretty clear now what the trouble is.'

'Really? Then what . . . ?'

'It's copper deficiency.' I said it casually as though I had been turning such a thing over in my mind right from the beginning. 'You can tell by the loss of the pigment in the coat, especially around the eyes. In fact when you look at them you can see that a lot of them are a bit paler than normal.' I waved an airy hand in the general direction of the stirks.

Charlie nodded. 'Aye, by gaw, you're right. Ah thowt they'd gone a funny colour.'

'Can we cure it?' Mrs Dalby asked the inevitable question.

'Oh yes, I'm going straight back to the surgery now to make up a copper mixture and we'll dose the lot. And you'll have to repeat that every fortnight while they are out at grass. It's a bit of a nuisance, I'm afraid, but there's no other way. Can you do it?'

'Oh aye, we'll do it,' Charlie said.

And 'Oh aye, we'll do it,' little William echoed, sticking out his chest and strutting around aggressively as though he wanted to start catching the beasts right away.

The treatment had a spectacular effect. I didn't have the modern long-lasting copper injections at my disposal but the solution of copper sulphate which I concocted under the surgery tap at Skeldale House worked like magic. Within a few weeks that batch of stirks was capering, lively and fully fleshed, over those hillside fields. Not a single death, no lingering unthriftiness. It was as though the whole thing had never happened, as though the hand of doom had never hovered over not only the cattle but the little family of humans.

It had been a close thing and, I realised, only a respite. That little woman had a long hard fight ahead of her still.

I have always abhorred change of any kind but it pleases me to come forward twenty years and spectate at another morning in the kitchen at Prospect House. I was seated at the same little table picking a buttered scone from the same tray and wondering whether I should follow it with a piece of malt bread or one of the jam tarts.

Billy still smiled down from the mantelpiece and Mrs Dalby, hands clasped in front of her, was watching me, her head a little on one side, the same half smile curving her lips. The years had not altered her much; there was some grey in her hair but the little red, weathered face and the bright eyes were as I had always known them.

I sipped my tea and looked across at the vast bulk of William sprawled in his father's old chair, smiling his father's smile at me. There were about fifteen stones of William and I had just been watching him in action as he held a fully grown bullock's hind foot while I examined it. The animal had made a few attempts to kick but the discouragement on its face had been obvious as William's great hands effortlessly engulfed its fetlock and a corner of his wide shoulder span dug into its abdomen.

No, I couldn't expect William to be the same, nor Dennis and Michael clattering into the kitchen now in their heavy boots and moving over to the sink to wash their hands. They were six footers too with their father's high-shouldered easy slouching walk but without William's sheer bulk.

Their tiny mother glanced at them then up at the picture on the mantelpiece.

'It would have been our thirtieth anniversary today,' she said conversationally.

I looked up at her, surprised. She never spoke of such things and I didn't know how to answer. I couldn't very well say 'congratulations' when she had spent twenty of those years alone. She had never said a word about her long fight; and it had been a winning fight. She had bought the neighbouring farm lower down the Dale when old Mr Mason retired; it was a good farm with better land and William had lived there after his marriage and they ran the two places as one. Things were pretty good now with her three expert stocksmen sons eliminating the need for outside labour except old Charlie who still pottered around doing odd jobs.

'Yes, thirty years,' Mrs Dalby said, looking slowly round the room as though she was seeing it for the first time. Then she turned back and bent over me, her face serious.

'Mr Herriot,' she said, and I was sure that at last, on this special day, she was going to say something about the years of struggle, the nights of worry and tears, the grinding toil.

For a moment she rested her hand lightly on my shoulder and her eyes looked into mine.

'Mr Herriot, are you quite sure that tea is to your liking?'

10

Every professional visit has its beginning in a call, a summons from the client which can take varying forms. . . .

'This is Joe Bentley speaking,' said the figure on the surgery doorstep. It was an odd manner of address, made stranger by the fact that Joe was holding his clenched fist up by his jaw and staring vacantly past me.

''ello, 'ello,' Joe continued as though into space, and suddenly everything became clear. That was an imaginary telephone he was holding and he was doing his best to communicate with the vet; and not doing badly considering the innumerable pints of beer that were washing around inside him.

On market days the pubs stayed open from ten o'clock till five and Joe was one of the now extinct breed who took their chance to drink themselves almost insensible. The modern farmer may have a few drinks on market day but the old reckless intake is rare now.

In Darrowby it was confined to a group of hard-bitten characters, all of them elderly, so even then the custom was on the wane. But it wasn't uncommon to see them when they came to pay their bills, leaning helplessly against the surgery wall and pushing their cheque books wordlessly at us. Some of them still used a pony and trap and the old joke about the horse taking them home was illustrated regularly. One old chap kept an enormously powerful ancient car simply for the purpose of getting him home; even if he engaged top gear by mistake when he collapsed into the driver's seat the vehicle would still take off. Some didn't go home at all on market day but spent the night carousing and playing cards till dawn.

As I looked at Joe Bentley swaying on the step I wondered what his programme might be for the rest of the evening. He closed his eyes, held his fist close to his face, and spoke again.

'Hellow, who's there?' he asked in an affected telephone voice.

'Herriot speaking,' I replied. Clearly Joe wasn't trying to be funny. He was just a little confused. It was only right to co-operate with him. 'How are you, Mr Bentley?'

'Nicely, thank ye,' Joe answered solemnly, eyes still tightly closed. 'Are you very well?'

'I'm fine, thanks. Now what can I do for you?'

This seemed to floor him temporarily because he remained silent for several seconds, opening his eyes occasionally and squinting somewhere over my left shoulder with intense concentration. Then something seemed to click; he closed his eyes again, cleared his throat and recommenced.

'Will you come up to ma place? I've a cow wants cleansin'.'

'Do you want me to come tonight?'

Joe gave this serious thought, pursing his lips and scratching his ear with his free hand before answering.

'Nay, morning'll do. Goodbye and thank ye.' He replaced the phantom telephone carefully in its rest, swung round and made his way down the street with great dignity. He hardly staggered at all and there was something purposeful in his bearing which convinced me that he was heading back to the Red Bear. For a moment I thought he would fall outside Johnson's the iron-mongers but by the time he rounded the corner into the market place he was going so well that I felt sure he'd make it.

And I can remember Mr Biggins standing by the desk in our office, hands deep in his pockets, chin thrust forward stubbornly.

'I 'ave a cow gruntin' a bit.'

'Oh, right, we'll have a look at her.' I reached for a pen to write the visit in the book.

He shuffled his feet. 'Well ah don't know. She's maybe not as bad as all that.'

'Well, whatever you say ...'

'No,' he said. 'It's what you say – you're t'vet.'

'It's a bit difficult,' I replied. 'After all, I haven't seen her. Maybe I'd better pay you a visit.'

'Aye, that's all very fine, but it's a big expense. It's ten bob every time you fellers walk on to ma place and that's before you start. There's all t'medicines and everything on top.'

'Yes, I understand, Mr Biggins. Well, would you like to take something away with you? A tin of stomach powder, perhaps?'

'How do you know it's t'stomach?'

'Well I don't actually . . .'

'It might be summat else.'

'That's very true, but . . .'

'She's a right good cow, this,' he said with a touch of aggression. 'Paid fifty pun for her at Scarburn Market.'

'Yes, I'm sure she is. And consequently I really think she'd be worth a visit. I could come out this afternoon.'

There was a long silence. 'Aye, but it wouldn't be just one visit, would it? You'd be comin' again next day and maybe the one after that and before we knew we'd 'ave a clonkin' great bill.'

'Yes, I'm sorry, Mr Biggins, everything is so expensive these days.'

'Yes, by gaw!' He nodded vigorously. 'Sometimes it ud be cheaper to give you t'cow at t'end of it.'

'Well now, hardly that . . . but I do see your point.'

I spent a few moments in thought. 'How about taking a fever drink as well as the stomach powder? That would be safer.'

He gave me a long blank stare. 'But you still wouldn't be sure, would you?'

'No, not quite sure, not absolutely . . .'

'She could even 'ave a wire in 'er.'

'True, very true.'

'Well then, shoving medicines down her neck isn't goin' to do no good is it?'

'It isn't, you're right.'

'Ah don't want to lose this cow, tha knows!' he burst out truculently. 'Ah can't afford to lose 'er!'

'I realise that, Mr Biggins. That's why I feel I should see her – I did suggest that if you remember.'

He did not reply immediately and only the strain in his eyes and a faint twitching of a cheek muscle betrayed the inner struggle which was raging. When he finally spoke it was in a hoarse croak.

'Aye, well, it might be best . . . but . . . er we could mebbes leave 'er till mornin' and see how she is then.'

'That's a good idea.' I smiled in relief. 'You have a look at her first thing in the morning and give me a ring before nine if she's no better.'

My words seemed to deepen his gloom. 'But what if she doesn't last till mornin'?'

'Well of course there is that risk.'

'Not much good ringin' you if she's dead, is it?'

'That's true, of course.'

'Ah'd be ringin' Mallock the knacker man, wouldn't I?'

'Afraid so, yes . . .'

'Well that's no bloody use to me, gettin' five quid from Mallock for a good cow!'

'Mm, no . . . I can see how you feel.'

'Ah think a lot about this cow!'

'I'm sure you do.'

'It ud be a big loss for me.'

'Quite.'

Mr Biggins hunched his shoulders and glared at me belligerently. 'Well then what are you goin' to do about 'er?'

'Let's see.' I ran my fingers through my hair. 'Perhaps you could wait till tonight and see if she recovers and if she isn't right by say, eight o'clock you could let me know and I'd come out.'

'You'd come out then, would you?' he said slowly, narrowing his eyes.

I gave him a bright smile. 'That's right.'

'Aye, but last time you came out at night you charged extra, ah'm sure you did.'

'Well, probably,' I said, spreading my hands. 'That's usual in veterinary practices.'

'So we're worse off than afore, aren't we?'

'When you look at it like that . . . I suppose so . . .'

'Ah'm not a rich man, tha knows.'

'I realise that.'

'Takes me all ma time to pay t'ordinary bill without extras.'

'Oh I'm sure . . .'

'So that idea's a bad egg, ain't it ?'

'Seems like it . . . yes . . .' I lay back in my chair, feeling suddenly tired.

Mr Biggins glowered at me morosely but I wasn't going to be tempted into any further gambits. I gave him what I fancied was a neutral stare and I hoped it conveyed the message that I was open to suggestions but wasn't going to make any myself.

The silence which now blanketed the room seemed to be of a durable nature. Down at the end of the street the church clock tolled the quarter hour, far off in the market place a dog barked, Miss Dobson, the grocer's daughter, glided past the window on her bicycle but no word was uttered.

Mr Biggins, biting his lower lip, darting his eyes desperately from his feet to me and back again, was clearly at the end of his resources, and it came to me at last that I had to take a firm initiative.

'Mr Biggins,' I said. 'I've got to be on my way. I have a lot of calls and one of them is within a mile of your farm, so I shall see your cow around three o'clock.' I stood up to indicate that the interview was over.

The farmer gave me a hunted look. I had the feeling that he had been resigned to a long period of stalemate and this sudden attack had taken him out of his stride. He opened his mouth as though to speak then appeared to change his mind and turned to go. At the door he paused, raised his hand and looked at me beseechingly for a moment, then he sank his chin on his chest and left the room.

I watched him through the window and as he crossed the road he stopped half way in the street in the same indeterminate way, muttering to himself and glancing back at the surgery; and as he lingered there I grew anxious that he might be struck by a passing car, but at length he squared his shoulders and trailed slowly out of sight.

*　　*　　*

And sometimes it isn't easy to get a clear picture over the telephone . . .

'This is Bob Fryer.'

'Good morning, Herriot here.'

'Now then, one of me sows is bad.'

'Oh right, what's the trouble?'

A throaty chuckle. 'Ah, that's what ah want *you* to tell *me*!'

'Oh, I see.'

'Aye, ah wouldn't be ringin' you up if I knew what the trouble was, would I? Heh, heh, heh, heh!'

The fact that I had heard this joke about two thousand times interfered with my full participation in the merriment but I managed a cracked laugh in return.

'That's perfectly true, Mr Fryer. Well, why have you rung me?'

'Damn, I've told ye – to find out what the trouble is.'

'Yes, I understand that, but I'd like some details. What do you mean when you say she's bad?'

'Well, she's just a bit off it.'

'Quite, but could you tell me a little more?'

A pause. 'She's dowly, like.'

'Anything else?'

'No . . . no . . . she's a right poorly pig, though.'

I spent a few moments in thought. 'Is she doing anything funny?'

'Funny? Funny? Nay, there's nowt funny about t'job, I'll tell tha! It's no laughin' matter.'

'Well . . . er . . . let me put it this way. Why are you calling me out?'

'I'm calling ye out because you're a vet. That's your job, isn't it?'

I tried again. 'It would help if I knew what to bring with me. What are her symptoms?'

'Symptoms? Well, she's just off colour, like.'

'Yes, but what is she doing?'

'She's doin' nowt. That's what bothers me.'

'Let's see.' I scratched my head. 'Is she very ill?'

'I reckon hes's in bad fettle.'

'But would you say it was an urgent matter?'

Another long pause. 'Well, she's nobbut middlin'. She's not framin' at all.'

'Yes ... yes ... and how long has she been like this?'

'Oh, for a bit.'

'But how long exactly?'

'For a good bit.'

'But Mr Fryer, I want to know when she started these symptoms. How long has she been affected?'

'Oh ... ever since we got 'er.'

'Ah, and when was that?'

'Well, she came wi' the others ...'

11

It was going to take a definite effort of will to get out of the car. I had driven about ten miles from Darrowby, thinking all the time that the Dales always looked their coldest, not when they were covered with snow, but as now, when the first sprinkling streaked the bare flanks of the fells in bars of black and white like the ribs of a crouching beast. And now in front of me was the farm gate rattling on its hinges as the wind shook it.

The car, heaterless and draughty as it was, seemed like a haven in an uncharitable world and I gripped the wheel tightly with my woollen-gloved hands for a few moments before opening the door. The wind almost tore the handle from my fingers as I got out but I managed to crash the door shut before stumbling over the frozen mud to the gate. Muffled as I was in heavy coat and scarf pulled up to my ears I could feel the icy gusts biting at my face, whipping up my nose and hammering painfully into the air spaces in my head.

I had driven through and, streaming-eyed, was about to get back into the car when I noticed something unusual. There was a frozen pond just off the path and among the rime-covered rushes which fringed the dead opacity of the surface a small object stood out, shiny black.

I went over and looked closer. It was a tiny kitten, probably about six weeks old, huddled and immobile, eyes tightly closed. Bending down, I poked gently at the furry body. It must be dead; a morsel like this couldn't possibly survive in such cold ... but no, there was a spark of life because the mouth opened soundlessly for a second then closed.

Quickly I lifted the little creature and tucked it inside my coat. As I drove into the farmyard I called to the farmer who was carrying two buckets out of the calf house. 'I've got one of your kittens here, Mr Butler. It must have strayed outside.'

Mr Butler put down his buckets and looked blank. 'Kitten? We haven't got no kittens at present.'

I showed him my find and he looked more puzzled.

'Well that's a rum 'un, there's no black cats on this spot. We've all sorts o' colours but no black 'uns.'

'Well he must have come from somewhere else,' I said. 'Though I can't imagine anything so small travelling very far. It's rather mysterious.'

I held the kitten out and he engulfed it with his big, work-roughened hand.

'Poor little beggar, he's only just alive. I'll take him into t'house and see if the missus can do owt for him.'

In the farm kitchen Mrs Butler was all concern. 'Oh what a shame!' She smoothed back the bedraggled hair with one finger. 'And it's got such a pretty face.' She looked up at me. 'What is it, anyway, a him or a her?'

I took a quick look behind the hind legs. 'It's a Tom.'

'Right,' she said. 'I'll get some warm milk into him but first of all we'll give him the old cure.'

She went over to the fireside oven on the big black kitchen range, opened the door and popped him inside.

I smiled. It was the classical procedure when new-born lambs were found suffering from cold and exposure; into the oven they went and the results were often dramatic. Mrs Butler left the door partly open and I could just see the little black figure inside; he didn't seem to care much what was happening to him.

The next hour I spent in the byre wrestling with the hind feet of a cow. The cleats were overgrown and grossly misshapen and upturned, causing the animal to hobble along on her heels. My job was to pare and hack away the excess horn and my long held opinion that the hind feet of a cow were never meant to be handled by man was thoroughly confirmed. We had a rope round the hock and the leg pulled up over a beam in the roof but the leg still pistoned back and forth while I hung on till my teeth rattled. By the time I had finished the sweat was running into my eyes and I had quite forgotten the cold day outside.

Still, I thought, as I eased the kinks from my spine when I had finished, there were compensations. There was a satisfaction in the sight of the cow standing comfortably on two almost normal looking feet.

'Well that's summat like,' Mr Butler grunted. 'Come in the house and wash your hands.'

In the kitchen as I bent over the brown earthenware sink I kept glancing across at the oven.

Mrs Butler laughed. 'Oh he's still with us. Come and have a look.'

It was difficult to see the kitten in the dark interior but when I spotted him I put out my hand and touched him and he turned his head towards me.

'He's coming round,' I said. 'That hour in there has worked wonders.'

'Doesn't often fail.' The farmer's wife lifted him out. 'I think he's a little tough 'un.' She began to spoon warm milk into the tiny mouth. 'I reckon we'll have him lappin' in a day or two.'

'You're going to keep him, then?'

'Too true we are. I'm going to call him Moses.'

'Moses?'

'Aye, you found him among the rushes, didn't you?'

I laughed. 'That's right. It's a good name.'

*   *   *

I was on the Butler farm about a fortnight later for the ever-recurring job of 'cleansing' a cow and I kept looking around for Moses. Farmers rarely have their cats indoors and I thought that if the black kitten had survived he would have joined the feline colony around the buildings.

Farm cats have a pretty good time. They may not be petted or cosseted but it has always seemed to me that they lead a free, natural life. They are expected to catch mice but if they are not so inclined there is abundant food at hand; bowls of milk here and there and the dogs' dishes to be raided if anything interesting is left over. I had seen plenty of cats around today, some flitting nervously away, others friendly and purring. There was a tabby loping gracefully across the cobbles and a big tortoise-shell was curled on a bed of straw at the warm end of the byre; cats are connoisseurs of comfort. When Mr Butler went to fetch the hot water I had a quick look in the bullock house and a white Tom regarded me placidly from between the bars of a hay rack where he had been taking a siesta. But there was no sign of Moses.

I finished drying my arms and was about to make a casual reference to the kitten when Mr Butler handed me my jacket.

'Come round here with me if you've got a minute,' he said. 'I've got summat to show you.'

I followed him through the door at the end and across a passage into the long, low-roofed piggery. He stopped at a pen about half way down and pointed inside.

'Look 'ere,' he said.

I leaned over the wall and my face must have shown my astonishment because the farmer burst into a shout of laughter.

'That's summat new for you, isn't it?'

I stared unbelievingly down at a large sow stretched comfortably on her side, suckling a litter of about twelve piglets and right in the middle of the long pink row, furry black and incongruous, was Moses. He had a teat in his mouth and was absorbing his nourishment with the same rapt enjoyment as his smooth-skinned fellows on either side.

'What the devil . . . ?' I gasped.

Mr Butler was still laughing. 'I thought you'd never have seen anything like that before, I never have, any road.'

'But how did it happen?' I still couldn't drag my eyes away.

'It was the Missus's idea,' he replied. 'When she'd got the little youth lappin' milk she took him out to find a right warm spot for him in the buildings. She settled on this pen because the sow, Bertha, had just had a litter and I had a heater in and it was grand and cosy.'

I nodded. 'Sounds just right.'

'Well she put Moses and a bowl of milk in here,' the farmer went on, 'but the little feller didn't stay by the heater very long – next time I looked in he was round at t'milk bar.'

I shrugged my shoulders. 'They say you see something new every day at this game, but this is something I've never even heard of. Anyway, he looks well on it – does he actually live on the sow's milk or does he still drink from his bowl?'

'A bit of both, I reckon. It's hard to say.'

Anyway, whatever mixture Moses was getting he grew rapidly into a sleek, handsome animal with an unusually high gloss to his coat which may or may not have been due to the porcine element of his diet. I never went to the Butlers' without having a look in the pig pen. Bertha, his foster mother, seemed to find nothing unusual in this hairy intruder and pushed him around casually with pleased grunts just as she did with the rest of her brood.

Moses for his part appeared to find the society of the pigs very congenial. When the piglets curled up together and settled down for a sleep Moses would be somewhere in the heap and when his young colleagues were weaned at eight weeks he showed his attachment to Bertha by spending most of his time with her.

And it stayed that way over the years. Often he would be right inside the pen, rubbing himself happily along the comforting bulk of the sow, but I remember him best in his favourite place; crouching on the wall looking down perhaps meditatively on what had been his first warm home.

12

I was beginning to learn a few tricks of my own.

In my bachelor days those early morning rings at the door-bell used to start me galloping downstairs into the freezing passage in my pyjamas full of enthusiasm, in fact almost burst-ing with impatience to learn what the immediate future held for me. But marriage had maybe softened me. At any rate, a long run of sessions in my bare feet on the doorstep with the bracing Yorkshire air whistling round my ankles had persuaded me that this was an overrated pastime.

The trouble was that in those days there were very few tele-phones on the farms and many of the farmers used to cycle in to the surgery when they wanted the vet; and of course farmers are inclined to rise rather early; a lot of them seemed to think that around 7 a.m. was a good time.

I just had to alter my system and now when I heard that long jangling downstairs I crawled out from beside Helen, tiptoed over to the window and opened it. Our bed-sitter being at the front of the house I was able to push my head through a few inches of space and carry on long conversations while most of me stayed warmly inside.

But on this Sunday morning something was wrong. I had heard the ring, taken up my kneeling position on the floor and got my head through the window. But I couldn't see anybody.

'Hello!' I called.

''ellow!' came back the reply immediately. But there was nobody on the step.

'Hello!' I shouted.

''ellow!' a hearty bellow responded.

'Hello!' I bawled at the top of my voice. I still couldn't see a soul.

''ellow, 'ellow, 'ellow!' echoed a full-throated yell with just a touch of asperity in it.

This was ridiculous. I didn't feel up to another effort – my head was beginning to throb – so I pushed the sash up a few inches more and leaned further out into the street.

And as I gazed down over the long stretch of ivy-covered brick it became clear why I had been unable to see anybody on the step. A man with very bandy legs encased in brown leggings was leaning against the wall of the house; he was bent double and apparently hollering straight down at the ground. I was baffled at first then I realised that he was directing his cries down through the small iron grating which led to the cellar. There was a chute there where the coalman used to tip his bags.

From my new vantage point I was able to attract the man's attention and when he looked up I saw it was Mr Dawson of Highstones.

He grinned cheerfully, quite unabashed. 'Oh, you're there are you? I have a cow with a touch o' felon. Give us a call some time this morning will you?' He waved and was gone.

I returned thoughtfully to Helen's side. And as I tried to drop off to sleep again the strong impression kept pushing into my consciousness that Mr Dawson wouldn't have been at all surprised if I had popped my head up through the grating instead of the window. It seemed to me that he had accepted the fact that I dwelt somewhere in the grimy darkness at the bottom of that cleft. It lent weight to an idea that had been growing in my mind for some time; that farmers looked on vets as different beings. We weren't really people at all.

There was Mr Coates last week. He had got me out of bed at 3 a.m. to a farrowing and when I stumbled, eyes half closed, from the car he was standing outside the piggery holding a lamp.

'Well now, Mr Herriot,' he said brightly, 'were you in bed when ah phoned?'

I stared at the man. 'In bed? Where the heck do you think I'd be at three o'clock in the morning?'

'Well ah don't know.' Mr Coates looked a little confused. 'Ah thought you might be up studyin'.'

There it was again. Up studyin'! Did they really think a vet was a creature apart – a kind of troglodyte who lived in a cell with only his text books and instruments for company? He didn't have a social life, he required no sleep, he didn't even have to eat. This last point was a very real one; I have often noticed a certain puzzlement in a farmer's face when I said I'd be as quick as I could but I'd have to finish my dinner first; or a pregnant silence at the end of the phone when I said I was just starting my breakfast.

But the man who most blatantly ignored my nutritional requirements and actually seemed to be trying to sabotage them was Mr Grainger of Beckton. He was a fierce man in his sixties and he called to see me every Saturday evening at six o'clock. What made this particularly wearing was that Helen chose each Saturday to put on a sumptuous high tea. Maybe she wanted to remind me of my Scottish upbringing but she used to set before me things like herrings in oatmeal with mustard sauce or sole and chips or ham and eggs and fill in the spaces on the table with new-baked scones, pancakes, curd tarts, cherry cakes.

It was usually when I was half way through the first course that the bell rang and there, sure enough, was Mr Grainger glaring belligerently through the glass door. He would never come into the house. All he wanted was a ten minutes' discussion on the doorstep. At first I used to say, 'I'm just at my tea,' or something like that, or I'd go on chewing in an exaggerated manner and keep wiping my lips on a napkin until I realised I was wasting my time. Mr Grainger was only interested in me as an object to talk at.

I said he wanted a discussion but that was the wrong word; he just wanted to air his views. An insight into his character could be gained from the remarks of one of his neighbours who told me that the Beckton Farmers' Discussion Group had folded up because whenever Mr Grainger got up to speak all the other farmers walked out.

In any case it seemed to enliven his Saturday evening to hold me trapped there while he described the symptoms displayed by his livestock during the previous week. He never asked me for advice; he made it quite clear that he knew a lot better than me how to treat his animals, but he did want to tell me about it.

And he told me at great length, his hands clasped over his stick in front of him, his eyes fixed on mine in a hostile stare.

But nothing is wholly bad and I did reap some small recompense from observing his antics as he tried to illustrate his case histories with actions.

I can recall one Saturday when he was complaining bitterly that he had been swindled over a carthorse he had just purchased. He was a particularly stiff-jointed man and not cut out for portraying the lameness of horses, but he managed to give an astounding impression of stringhalt. I diagnosed it instantly as he strutted up and down the pavement in front of Skeldale House, jerking one leg up behind him at every step. Then he stopped abruptly and held the offending limb out, quivering, behind him . . . good heavens, maybe he was a shiverer, too! The farmer kept his eyes on me and seemed oblivious of the interest of the passers-by. There were quite a few people in the street, probably bound for the early show at the cinema, but for the moment they appeared to find Mr Grainger more entertaining.

'And that's not all,' he cried. 'There's summat wrang with his watterworks.'

'Really? How do you mean?'

'Why 'e can't stale properly. Has a 'ell of a job. Gets himself all wraxed up like this.'

Mr Grainger went into another of his impersonations – that of a horse having difficulty in passing urine – and I had to admit it was probably his best yet. He planted his stick firmly on the pavement and holding the top with both hands he backed away from it till his body was parallel with the ground. Then he began to straddle his legs further and further apart. The knot of people on the other side of the road had increased to a fair-sized crowd and they stared, fascinated, at the extraordinary sight. Mr Grainger was indeed the very picture of equine suffering and as he hollowed his back and paddled his wide-spaced feet I could almost share the desperate battle for release. When he finally raised his head and groaned the effect was harrowing.

When all was finished Mr Grainger did as he always did –

gave me a cold nod and stumped off without a word. There was no need for him to say, 'See you next Saturday'. I knew he'd be back.

Then there was Mr Grimsdale. His attitude towards me was something I couldn't quite make out, but I did know that he always had a depressing effect on me. He did this by the simple expedient of telling me that I didn't look very well.

I thought back to the visit to his farm yesterday when he had called me to a cow with a cut teat. He was a tall cadaverous man with sunken cheeks and a mournful expression – he would have made a wonderful undertaker – and he looked at me in his own particular way as I got out of the car.

I wondered what it would be today. My own conviction is that you should never tell anybody they don't look well, no matter what you think. And Mr Grimsdale's little sallies bit especially deeply because he always referred to me in agricultural terms as though I were one of his bullocks.

'You've lost a bit o' ground lately, young man,' he would say, directing a piercing glance from my face down to my feet and down again. 'Aye, you're losin' ground fast – it's plain to see.'

Or another time it might be, 'You've run off a bit, Mr Herriot. There's no doubt you've run off.' And his stick would twitch in his hand as if he would have liked to give me an exploratory poke.

But today he didn't say anything until I had finished stitching the teat and was washing my hands in a bucket of water. Then as I straightened up he adopted his usual stance; throwing up his head and jutting his chin he appraised me gloomily.

'You've failed since ah last saw you, young man. Soon as you walked across t'yard this morning ah thought to meself, aye that lad's failed over t'last week or two.'

And as the sharp eyes bored into me from behind the long pointed nose his viewpoint was plain. He, at any rate, could contemplate the prospect of my early demise with some compassion but without going to pieces.

I worked up a sickly smile as I always did.

'Oh, I'm fine, Mr Grimsdale, never felt better.' But the voice had an uncertain quaver and I knew by my sinking stomach that his shaft had gone home again. And then there was the usual humiliating business when I had driven away. I always stopped the car just round the corner where a high curve of wall hid me from the farm.

Staring into the car mirror I put out my tongue, pulled down my eyelids to have a look at my mucous membranes and muttered desperately as though Mr Grimsdale was still there.

'I feel fine, really I do ... fine ... fine ...'

Talking of farmers' attitudes to their vets, I think it is fair to say that in Robert Hewison's cheerful household, though Siegfried's prowess as an animal doctor was highly regarded, his main claim to fame was as a judge of Christmas cake.

Mrs Hewison was a baker of great repute and when she started long before the festive season to stir up vast quantities of fruit and candied peel and butter and all the other things that went into her peerless cakes it was a very serious business. Not that there was any question of a failure – her cakes varied from excellent to superb – but once the long process had been completed and the last piece of marzipan and icing applied she dearly loved to have the accolade from an expert. And in her eyes Siegfried was number one.

Robert Hewison confided in me once: 'Tha knows, my missus is never content till your guvnor's had a taste.'

I was privileged to be present on one of these occasions. It was a few days before Christmas and Siegfried and I had gone together to Robert's farm to lift a horse which had got cast in its stall. We did the job successfully with the aid of slings and a block and tackle and Robert, as always, asked us into the house.

The farmer's wife, her dark, rather solemn face illumined by friendly eyes, ushered us to the two tall wooden chairs by the fireside.

'Come and get warmed up, gentlemen,' she said. 'And you'll have a drink and a bit o' cake, won't you?'

'You're very kind, Mrs Hewison,' replied Siegfried. 'That would be lovely.'

He sat down, but I went through to the offshoot of the kitchen to wash my hands at the sink. The farmer's wife was cutting at a large cake on a table nearby. She nudged me and whispered conspiratorially.

'This isn't me own cake. It's one me sister baked, but I'm not telling Mr Farnon that. We'll just see what he says.'

I stared at her. 'But is that quite fair? Hadn't you better tell him?'

'No, I want to have his true judgement, so I'm not sayin' a word.'

I went back to the kitchen with some misgiving. It was unlike this lady to play jokes, but maybe after years of unqualified approbation she wanted to put my colleague's sincerity to the test. Anyway, I hoped nothing unfortunate would happen.

As I took my place by the fire Robert and his three sons came in and sat around in a circle. I was given a piece of cake, too, but nobody paid any attention to me; all eyes were on Siegfried.

'I'd like to know what you think of t'cake this year, Mr Farnon,' our hostess said.

My colleague toasted the family gracefully, sipped at his whisky then lifted the plate with its slice of cake. Silence fell upon the company. Holding the plate in the palm of his hand he studied the cake carefully from various angles before breaking off a fair-sized piece. This he massaged gently between thumb and forefinger for a few moments, his eyes half closed. Then after sniffing at it a couple of times he put it in his mouth.

I could feel the tension building in the room as he chewed gravely, his face quite expressionless. When he had finally swallowed the portion he smacked his lips once or twice meditatively then turned his head and looked full at Mrs Hewison. Amid a deathly hush they gazed into each other's eyes for several long seconds but Siegfried still didn't say anything. Instead he reached for his glass again and took another drink of whisky which he seemed to wash around his mouth before breaking off another portion of cake.

He took a long time over this piece, chewing in a slow motion, his eyes, deadly serious, staring sightlessly in front of him. Robert, the boys, all of us, leaned a little forward in our chairs, as he finally swallowed the last crumb, wiped his lips and sat immobile, apparently wrapped in thought. Then as he clearly came to a decision he sat upright in his chair, straightened his shoulders and turned resolutely towards the lady of the house once more.

Siegfried was and is a man of the highest principle. Over the years I have known him he has always given his opinions truthfully, fearlessly and with a total disregard of the consequences; and though this trait ruffled the stream of his life on occasion, there were times, as now, when it stood him in good stead.

'Mrs Hewison,' he said, his eyes steady and unwavering. 'This is a good cake.' He paused. 'A very good cake indeed.' He hesitated again and I could see the real iron in the man coming out. 'But if you will permit me, I'm bound to say that it is not up to your usual standard.'

Mrs Hewison, usually an undemonstrative person, burst into a loud cry of delight and Robert and his sons, who were obviously in on the joke, roared and clapped their hands.

Siegfried looked around in some surprise at the sudden tumult which went on and on as though somebody had scored a goal in the cup final. He was obviously puzzled and of course there was no way he could know that his previous exalted position in the household was now utterly impregnable.

13

I was back at Granville Bennett's again. Back in the tiled operating theatre with the great lamp pouring its harsh light over my colleague's bowed head, over the animal nurses, the rows of instruments, the little animal stretched on the table.

Until late this afternoon I had no idea that another visit to Hartington was in store for me; not until the doorbell rang as I was finishing a cup of tea and I went along the passage and opened the door and saw Colonel Bosworth on the step. He was holding a wicker cat basket.

'Can I trouble you for a moment, Mr Herriot?' he said.

His voice sounded different and I looked up at him questioningly. Most people had to look up at Colonel Bosworth with his lean six feet three inches and his tough soldier's face which matched the D.S.O. and M.C. which he had brought out of the war. I saw quite a lot of him, not only when he came to the surgery but out in the country where he spent most of his time hacking along the quiet roads around Darrowby on a big hunter with two Cairn terriers trotting behind. I liked him. He was a formidable man but he was unfailingly courteous and there was a gentleness in him which showed in his attitude to his animals.

'No trouble,' I replied. 'Please come inside.'

In the waiting room he held out the basket. His eyes were strained and there was shock and hurt in his face.

'It's little Maudie,' he said.

'Maudie . . . your black cat?' When I had been to his house the little creature had usually been in evidence, rubbing down the colonel's ankles, jumping on his knee competing assiduously with the terriers for his attention.

'What's the matter, is she ill?'

'No . . . no . . .' He swallowed and spoke carefully. 'She's had an accident, I'm afraid.'

'What kind of accident?'

'A car struck her. She never goes out into the road in front of the house but for some reason she did this afternoon.'

'I see.' I took the basket from him. 'Did the wheel go over her?'

'No, I don't think it can have done that because she ran back into the house afterwards.'

'Oh well,' I said. 'That sounds hopeful. It probably isn't anything very much.'

The colonel paused for a moment. 'Mr Herriot, I wish you were right but its ... rather frightful. It's her face you see. Must have been a glancing blow but I ... really don't see how she can live.'

'Oh ... as bad as that ... I'm sorry. Anyway come through with me and I'll have a look.'

He shook his head. 'No, I'll stay here if you don't mind. And there's just one thing.' He laid his hand briefly on the basket. 'If you think, as I do, that it's hopeless, please put her to sleep immediately. She must not suffer any more.'

I stared at him uncomprehendingly for a moment then hurried along the passage to the operating room. I put the basket on the table, slid the wooden rod from its loops and opened the lid. I could see the sleek little black form crouched in the depths and as I stretched my hand out gingerly towards it the head rose slowly and turned towards me with a long, open-mouthed wail of agony.

And it wasn't just an open mouth. The whole lower jaw was dangling uselessly, the mandible shattered and splintered, and as another chilling cry issued from the basket I had a horrific glimpse of jagged ends of bone gleaming from the froth of blood and saliva.

I closed the basket quickly and leaned on the lid.

'Christ!' I gasped. 'Oh Christ!'

I closed my eyes but couldn't dispel the memory of the grotesque face, the terrible sound of pain and worst of all the eyes filled with the terrified bewilderment which makes animal suffering so unbearable.

With trembling haste I reached behind me to the trolley for the bottle of Nembutal. This was the one thing vets could do, at any rate; cut short this agony with merciful speed. I pulled 5 c.c.'s into the syringe; more than enough – she'd drift into sleep and never wake up again. Opening the basket I reached down and underneath the cat and slipped the needle through the abdominal skin; an intraperitoneal injection would have to do. But as I depressed the plunger it was as though a calmer and less involved person was tapping me on the shoulder and saying, 'Just a minute, Herriot, take it easy. Why don't you think about this for a bit?'

I stopped after injecting 1 c.c. That would be enough to anaesthetise Maudie. In a few minutes she would feel nothing. Then I closed the lid and began to walk about the room. I had repaired a lot of cats' broken jaws in my time; they seemed to be prone to this trouble and I had gained much satisfaction from wiring up symphyseal fractures and watching their uneventful healing. But this was different.

After five minutes I opened the basket and lifted the little cat, sound asleep and as limp as a rag doll, on to the table.

I swabbed out the mouth and explored with careful fingers, trying to piece the grisly jigsaw together. The symphysis had separated right enough and that could be fastened together with wire, but how about those mandibular rami, smashed clean through on both sides – in fact there were two fractures on the left. And some of the teeth had been knocked out and others slackened; there was nothing to get hold of. Could they be held together by metal plates screwed into the bone? Maybe . . . and was there a man with the skill and equipment to do such a job . . . ? I thought I just might know one.

I went over the sleeping animal carefully; there wasn't a thing amiss except that pathetic drooping jaw. Meditatively I stroked the smooth, shining fur. She was only a young cat with years of life in front of her and as I stood there the decision came to me with a surge of relief and I trotted back along the passage to ask the colonel if I could take Maudie through to Granville Bennett.

It had started to snow heavily when I set out and I was glad it was downhill all the way to Hartington; many of the roads higher up the Dale would soon be impassable on a night like this.

In the Veterinary Hospital I watched the big man drilling, screwing, stitching. It wasn't the sort of job which could be hurried but it was remarkable how quickly those stubby fingers could work. Even so, we had been in the theatre for nearly an hour and Granville's complete absorption showed in the long silences broken only by the tinkling of instruments, occasional barking commands and now and then a sudden flare of exasperation. And it wasn't only the nurses who suffered; I had scrubbed up and had been pressed into service and when I failed to hold the jaw exactly as my colleague desired he exploded in my face.

'Not that bloody way, Jim! . . . What the hell are you playing at ? . . . No, no, no, no, *no*! . . . . . Oh God Almighty!'

But at last all was finished and Granville threw off his cap and turned away from the table with the air of finality which had made me envy him the first time. He was sweating. In his office he washed his hands, towelled his brow, and pulled on an elegant grey jacket from the pocket of which he produced a pipe. It was a different pipe from last time; I learned in time that all Granville's pipes were not only beautiful but big and this one had a bowl like a fair-sized coffee cup. He rubbed it gently along the side of his nose, gave it a polish with the yellow cloth he always seemed to carry and held it lovingly against the light.

'Straight grain, Jim. Superb, isn't it ?'

He contentedly scooped tobacco from his vast pouch, ignited it and puffed a cloud of delectable smoke at me before taking me by the arm. 'Come on, laddie. I'll show you round while they're clearing up in there.'

We did a tour of the hospital, taking in the waiting and consulting rooms, X-ray room, dispensary and, of course, the office with its impressive card index system with case histories of all patients, but the bit I enjoyed most was walking along the row of heated cubicles where an assortment of animals were recovering from their operations.

Granville stabbed his pipe at them as we went along. 'Spay, enterotomy, aural haematoma, entropion.' Then he bent suddenly, put a finger through the wire front and adopted a wheedling tone. 'Come now, George, come on little fellow, don't be frightened, it's only Uncle Granville.'

A small West Highland with a leg in a cast hobbled to the front and my colleague tickled his nose through the wire.

'That's George Wills-Fentham,' he said in explanation. 'Old Lady Wills-Fentham's pride and joy. Nasty compound fracture but he's doing very nicely. He's a bit shy is George but a nice little chap when you get to know him, aren't you, old lad ?' He continued his tickling and in the dim light I could see the short white tail wagging furiously.

Maudie was lying in the very last of the recovery pens, a tiny, trembling figure. That trembling meant she was coming out of the anaesthetic and I opened the door and stretched my hand out to her. She still couldn't raise her head but she was looking at me and as I gently stroked her side, her mouth opened in a faint rusty miaow. And with a thrill of deep pleasure I saw that her lower jaw belonged to her again; she could open and close it; that hideous dangling tatter of flesh and bone was only a bad memory.

'Marvellous, Granville,' I murmured. 'Absolutely bloody marvellous.'

Smoke plumed in quiet triumph from the noble pipe. 'Yes, it's not bad, is it laddie. A week or two on fluids and she'll be as good a new. No problems there.'

I stood up. 'Great! I can't wait to tell Colonel Bosworth. Can I take her home tonight ?'

'No, Jim, no. Not this time. I just want to keep an eye on her for a couple of days then maybe the colonel can collect her himself.' He led me back into the brightly lit office where he eyed me for a moment.

'You must come and have a word with Zoe while you're here,' he said. 'But first, just a suggestion. I wonder if you'd care to slip over with me to . . .'

I took a rapid step backward. 'Well . . . er . . . really. I don't think so,' I gabbled. 'I enjoyed my visit to the club that other night but . . . er . . . perhaps not this evening.'

'Hold on, laddie, hold on,' Granville said soothingly. 'Who said anything about the club ? No, I just wondered if you'd like to come to a meeting with me ?'

'Meeting ?'

'Yes, Professor Milligan's come through from Edinburgh to speak to the Northern Veterinary Society about metabolic diseases. I think you'd enjoy it.'

'You mean milk fever, acetonaemia and all that?'

'Correct. Right up your street, old son.'

'Well it is, isn't it? I wonder . . .' I stood for a few moments deep in thought, and one of the thoughts was why an exclusively small animal man like Granville wanted to hear about cow complaints. But I was maybe doing him an injustice; he probably wanted to maintain a broad, liberal view of veterinary knowledge.

It must have been obvious that I was dithering because he prodded me a little further.

'I'd like to have your company, Jim, and anyway I see you're all dressed and ready for anything. Matter of fact when you walked in tonight I couldn't help thinking what a smart lad you looked.'

He was right there. I hadn't dashed through in my farm clothes this time. With the memory of my last visit still painfully fresh in my mind I was determined that if I was going to meet the charming Zoe again I was going to be: (a) Properly dressed, (b) Sober, (c) in a normal state of health and not bloated and belching like an impacted bullock. Helen, agreeing that my image needed refurbishing, had rigged me out in my best suit.

Granville ran his hand along my lapel. 'Fine piece of serge if I may say so.'

I made up my mind. 'Right, I'd like to come with you. Just let me ring Helen to say I won't be straight back and then I'm your man.'

14

Outside it was still snowing; city snow drifting down in a wet curtain which soon lost itself in the dirty churned-up slush in the streets. I pulled my coat higher round my neck and huddled deeper in the Bentley's leather luxury. As we swept past dark buildings and shops I kept expecting Granville to turn up some side street and stop, but within a few minutes we were speeding through the suburbs up towards the North Road. This meeting, I thought, must be out in one of the country institutes, and I didn't say anything until we had reached Scotch Corner and the big car had turned on to the old Roman Road at Bowes.

I stretched and yawned. 'By the way, Granville, where are they holding this meeting?'

'Appleby,' my colleague replied calmly.

I came bolt upright in my seat then I began to laugh.

'What's the joke, old son?' Granville enquired.

'Well ... Appleby ... ha-ha-ha! Come on, where are we really heading?'

'I've told you, laddie, the Pemberton Arms, Appleby, to be exact.'

'Do you mean it?'

'Of course.'

'But hell, Granville, that's on the other side of the Pennines.'

'Quite right. Always has been, laddie.'

I ran a hand through my hair. 'Wait a minute. Surely it isn't worth going about forty miles in weather like this. We'll never get over Bowes Moor you know – in fact I heard yesterday it was blocked. Anyway, it's nearly eight o'clock – we'd be too late.'

The big man reached across and patted my knee.

'Stop worrying, Jim. We'll get there and we'll be in plenty of time. You've got to remember you're sitting in a proper motor car now. A drop of snow is nothing.'

As if determined to prove his word he put his foot down and the great car hurtled along the dead straight stretch of road. We skidded a bit on the corner at Greta Bridge then roared through Bowes and up to the highest country. I couldn't see much. In fact on the moor top I couldn't see anything, because up there it was the real country snow; big dry flakes driving straight into the headlights and settling comfortably with millions of their neighbours on the already deep white carpet on the road. I just didn't know how Granville was able to see, never mind drive fast; and I had no idea how we were going to get back over here in a few hours' time when the wind had drifted the snow across the road. But I kept my mouth shut. It was becoming increasingly obvious that I emerged as a sort of maiden aunt in Granville's company, so I held my peace and prayed.

I followed this policy through Brough and along the lower road where the going was easier until I climbed out with a feeling of disbelief in the yard of the Pemberton Arms. It was nine o'clock.

We slipped into the back of the room and I settled into my chair, prepared to improve my mind a little. There was a man on the platform holding forth and at first I had difficulty in picking up the substance of his words; he wasn't mentioning anything about animal diseases but suddenly everything clicked into place.

'We are indeed grateful,' the man was saying, 'to Professor Milligan for coming all this way and for giving us a most interesting and instructive talk. I know I speak for the entire audience when I say we have enjoyed it thoroughly, so may I ask you to show your appreciation in the usual manner.' There was a long round of applause then an outburst of talk and a pushing back of chairs.

I turned to Granville in some dismay. 'That was the vote of thanks. It's finished.'

'So it is, laddie.' My colleague didn't seem unduly disappointed or even surprised. 'But come with me – there are compensations.'

We joined the throng of vets and moved across the richly carpeted hall to another room where bright lights shone down on a row of tables laden with food. Then I recognised Bill Warrington the Burroughs Wellcome representative and all became clear.

This was a commercially sponsored evening and the real action, in Granville's estimation, began right here. I remembered then that Siegfried had once told me that Granville hated to miss any of these occasions. Though the most generous of men there was some piquancy in the gratis food and drink which attracted him irresistibly.

Even now he was guiding me purposefully towards the bar. But our progress was slow due to a phenomenon peculiar to Granville; everybody seemed to know him. Since those days I have been with him to restaurants, pubs, dances and it has been just the same. In fact I have often thought that if I took him to visit some lost tribe in the jungles of the Amazon one of them would jump and say, 'Well hello, Granville old boy!' and slap him on the back.

Finally however he fought his way through his fellow vets and we reached the bar where two dark little men in white coats were already under pressure; they were working with the impersonal concentration of people who knew that the whisky always took a hammering on veterinary evenings, but they paused and smiled as my colleague's massive presence hovered at the counter.

'Now then, Mr Bennett. How are you, Mr Bennett ?'

'Good evening, Bob. Nice to see you, Reg.' Granville responded majestically.

I noticed that Bob put down his bottle of ordinary whisky and reached down for a bottle of Glenlivet Malt to charge Granville's glass. The big man sniffed the fine spirit appreciatively.

'And one for my friend, Mr Herriot,' he said.

The barmen's respectful expressions made me feel suddenly important and I found myself in possession of my own vast measure of Glenlivet. I had to get it down quickly followed by a few speedy refills since the barmen took their cue from my companion's consumption.

Then I followed in Granville's regal wake as he made his way among the tables with the air of a man in his natural environment. Messrs Burroughs Wellcome had done us proud and we worked our way through a variety of canapes, savouries and cold meats. Now and again we revisited the bar for more of the Glenlivet then back to the tables.

I knew I had drunk too much and now I was eating too much.

But the difficulty with Granville was that if I ever declined anything he took it as a personal insult.

'Try one of those prawn things,' he would say, sinking his teeth into a mushroom vol au vent and if I hesitated a wounded look would come into his eyes.

But I was enjoying myself. Veterinary surgeons are my favourite people and I revelled as I always did in their tales of successes and failures. Especially the failures; they were particularly soothing. Whenever the thought of how we were going to get home stole into my mind I banished it quickly.

Granville seemed to have no qualms because he showed no signs of moving when the company began to thin out; in fact we were the last to leave, our departure being accorded a touch of ceremony by a final substantial stirrup cup from Bob and Reg.

As we left the hotel I felt fine; a little light-headed perhaps and with the merest hint of regret at being pressed to a second helping of trifle and cream, but otherwise in excellent shape. As we settled once more into the Bentley Granville was at his most expansive.

'Excellent meeting that, Jim. I told you it would be worth the journey.'

We were the only members of the company who were headed eastward and were alone on the road. In fact it occurred to me that we hadn't seen a single car on the road to Appleby and now there was something uncomfortable in our total isolation. The snow had stopped and the brilliant moon flooded its cold light over a white empty world. Empty, that is, except for us, and our solitary state was stressed by the smooth, virgin state of the glistening carpet ahead.

I was conscious of an increasing disquiet as the great gaunt spine of the Pennines bulked before us and as we drew nearer it reared up like an angry white monster.

Past the snow-burdened roofs of Brough then the long climb with the big car slipping from side to side as it fought its way up the bending, twisting hill, engine bellowing. I thought I'd feel better when we reached the top but the first glimpse of the

Bowes Moor road sent my stomach into a lurch of apprehension; miles and miles of it coiling its way across the most desolate stretch of country in all England. And even from this distance you could see the drifts, satin smooth and beautiful, pushing their deadly way across our path.

On either side of the road a vast white desert rolled and dipped endlessly toward the black horizon; there was not a light, not a movement, not a sign of life anywhere.

The pipe jutted aggressively as Granville roared forward to do battle. We hit the first drift, slewed sideways for a tense few seconds then we were on the other side, speeding into the unbroken surface. Then the next drift and the next and the next. Often I thought we were stuck but always, wheels churning, engine screaming we emerged. I had had plenty of experience of snow driving and I could appreciate Granville's expertise as, without slackening speed he picked out the shallowest, narrowest part of each obstruction for his attack. He had this heavy powerful car to help him but he could drive all right.

However, my trepidation at being stranded in this waste land was gradually being overshadowed by another uneasiness. When I had left the hotel I was pretty well topped up with food and drink and if I had been handled gently for the next few hours I'd have been all right. But on the bumpy journey to Brough I had been increasingly aware of a rising queasiness; my mind kept flitting back unhappily to that exotic cocktail, Reg's speciality, which Granville had said I must try; he had prevailed on me too, to wash down the whiskies with occasional beers which, he said, were essential to maintain a balanced intake of fluids and solids. And that final trifle – it had been a mistake.

And now I wasn't just being bumped, I was being thrown around like a pea in a drum as the Bentley lurched and skidded and occasionally took off altogether. Soon I began to feel very ill indeed. And like a seasick man who didn't care if the ship foundered I lost all interest in our progress; I closed my eyes, braced my feet on the floor and shrunk into an inner misery.

I hardly noticed as, after an age of violent motion, we finally began to go downhill and thundered through Bowes. After that there was little danger of having to spend the night in the car but Granville kept his foot down and we rocked over the frozen ground while I felt steadily worse.

I would dearly have loved to ask my colleague to stop and allow me to be quietly sick by the roadside but how do you say such a thing to a man who never seemed to be in the least affected by over-indulgence and who, even at that moment was chatting gaily as he refilled his pipe with his free hand. The internal pounding seemed to have forced extra alcohol into my bloodstream because on top of my other discomforts my vision was blurred, I was dizzy and had the strong conviction that if I tried to stand up I would fall flat on my face.

I was busy with these preoccupations when the car stopped. 'We'll just pop in and say hello to Zoe,' Granville said.

'Wha's that?' I slurred.

'We'll go inside for a few minutes.'

I looked around. 'Where are we?'

Granville laughed. 'Home, old son. I can see a light, so Zoe's still up. You must come and have a quick cup of coffee.'

I crawled laboriously from the seat and stood leaning on the car. My colleague tripped lightly to the door and rang the bell. He was as fit as a fiddle I thought bitterly as I reeled after him. I was slumped against the porch breathing heavily when the door opened and there was Zoe Bennett, bright eyed, glowing, beautiful as ever.

'Why Mr Herriot!' she cried. 'How nice to see you again!'

Slack-jawed, green-faced, rumple-suited, I stared into her eyes, gave a gentle hiccup and staggered past her into the house.

Next morning Granville rang to say all was going to be well because Maudie had been able to lap a little milk. It was kind of him to let me know and I didn't want to sound churlish by saying that was all I had managed to do, too.

It happened that morning by a coincidence that I had a far outlying visit and had to pass the Scotch Corner turning on the North Road. I stopped the car and sat gazing at the long snow-covered road stretching towards the Pennines. I was starting my engine when an A.A. man came over and spoke at my window.

'You're not thinking of trying the Bowes Moor road, are you?' he said.

'No, no. I was just looking.'

He nodded in satisfaction.

'I'm glad to hear that. It's blocked you know. There hasn't been a car over there for two days.'

15

One of the things Helen and I had to do was furnish our bed-sitter and kitchen. And when I say 'furnish' I use the word in its most austere sense. We had no high-flown ideas about luxury; it was, after all, a temporary arrangement and anyway we had no money to throw around.

My present to Helen at the time of our marriage was a modest gold watch and this had depleted my capital to the extent that a bank statement at the commencement of our married life revealed the sum of twenty-five shillings standing to my credit. Admittedly I was a partner now but when you start from scratch it takes a long time to get your head above water.

But we did need the essentials like a table, chairs, cutlery, crockery, the odd rug and carpet, and Helen and I decided that it would be most sensible to pick up these things at house sales. Since I was constantly going round the district I was able to drop in at these events and the duty of acquiring our necessities had been delegated to me. But after a few weeks it was clear that I was falling down on the job.

I had never realised it before but I had a blind spot in these matters. I would go to a sale and come away with a pair of brass candlesticks and a stuffed owl. On another occasion I acquired an ornate inkwell with a carved metal figure of a dog on it to-gether with a polished wooden box with innumerable fascinating little drawers and compartments for keeping homeopathic prescriptions. I could go on for a long time about the things I bought but they were nearly all useless.

Helen was very nice about it.

'Jim,' she said one day when I was proudly showing her a model of a fully rigged sailing ship in a bottle which I had been lucky enough to pick up, 'it's lovely, but I don't think we need it right now.'

I must have been a big disappointment to the poor girl and also to the local auctioneers who ran the sales. These gentlemen, when they saw me hovering around the back of the crowd would cheer up visibly. They, in common with most country folk, thought all vets were rich and that I would be bidding for some of the more expensive items. When a nice baby grand piano came up they would look over the heads at me with an expectant smile and their disappointment was evident when I finally went away with a cracked-faced barometer or a glove stretcher.

A sense of my failure began to seep through to me and when I had to take a sample through to the Leeds laboratory I saw a chance to atone.

'Helen,' I said, 'there's a huge saleroom right in the city centre. I'll take an hour off and go in there. I'm bound to see something we need.'

'Oh good!' my wife replied. 'That's a great idea! There'll be lots to choose from there. You haven't had much chance to find anything at those country sales.' Helen was always kind.

After my visit to the Leeds lab I asked the way to the sale-rooms.

'Leave your car here,' one of the locals advised me. 'You'll never park in the main street and you can get a tram right to the door.'

I was glad I listened to him because when I arrived the traffic was surging both ways in a nonstop stream. The saleroom was at the top of an extraordinarily long flight of smooth stone steps leading right to the top of the building. When I arrived, slightly out of breath, I thought immediately I had come to the right place, a vast enclosure strewn with furniture, cookers, gramophones, carpets – everything you could possibly want in a house.

I wandered around fascinated for quite a long time then my attention centred on two tall piles of books quite near to where the auctioneer was selling. I lifted one of them. It was *The Geography of the World*. I had never seen such beautiful books; as big as encyclopaedias and with thick embossed covers and gold lettering. The pages, too, were edged with gold and the paper was of a delightfully smooth texture. Quite enthralled I turned the pages, marvelling at the handsome illustrations, the coloured pictures each with its covering transparent sheet. They were a little old-fashioned, no doubt, and when I looked at the front I saw they were printed in 1858; but they were things of beauty.

Looking back, I feel that fate took a hand here because I had just reluctantly turned away when I heard the auctioneer's voice.

'Now then, here's a lovely set of books. *The Geography of the World in Twenty Four Volumes*. Just look at them. You don't find books like them today. Who'll give me a bid?'

I agreed with him. They were unique. But they must be worth pounds. I looked round the company but nobody said a word.

'Come on, ladies and gentlemen, surely somebody wants this wonderful addition to their library. Now what do I hear?'

Again the silence than a seedy looking man in a soiled mackintosh spoke up.

'Arf a crown,' he said morosely.

I looked around expecting a burst of laughter at this sally, but nobody was amused. In fact the auctioneer didn't seem surprised.

'I have a half a crown bid.' He glanced about him and raised his hammer. With a thudding of the heart I realised he was going to sell.

I heard my own voice, slightly breathless. 'Three shillings.'

'I have a bid of three shillings for *The Geography of the World in Twenty Four Volumes.* Are you all done?' Bang went the hammer. 'Sold to the gentleman over there.'

They were mine! I couldn't believe my luck. This surely was the bargain to end all bargains. I paid my three shillings while one of the men tied a length of rough string round each pile. The first pause in my elation came when I tried to lift my purchases. Books are heavy things and these were massive specimens; and there were twenty-four of them.

With a hand under each string I heaved like a weight-lifter and, pop-eyed, veins standing out on my forehead, I managed to get them off the ground and began to stagger shakily to the exit.

The first string broke on the top step and twelve of my volumes cascaded downwards over the smooth stone. After the first moment of panic I decided that the best way was to transport the intact set down to the bottom and come back for the others. I did this but it took me some time and I began to perspire before I was all tied up again and poised on the kerb ready to cross the road.

The second string broke right in the middle of the tramlines as I attempted a stiff-legged dash through a break in the traffic. For about a year I scrabbled there in the middle of the road while horns hooted, tram bells clanged and an interested crowd watched from the sidewalks. I had just got the escaped volumes in a column and was reknotting the string when the other lot burst from their binding and slithered gently along the metal rails; and it was when I was retrieving them that I noticed a large policeman, attracted by the din and the long line of vehicles, walking with measured strides in my direction.

In my mental turmoil I saw myself for the first time in the hands of the law. I could be done on several charges – Breach of the Peace, Obstructing Traffic to name only two – but I perceived that the officer was approaching very slowly and rightly or wrongly I feel that when a policeman strolls towards you like that he is a decent chap and is giving you a chance to get away. I took my chance. He was still several yards off when I had my two piles reassembled and I thrust my hands under the strings, tottered to the far kerb and lost myself in the crowd.

When I finally decided there was no longer any fear of feeling the dread grip on my shoulder I stopped in my headlong flight and rested in a shop doorway. I was puffing like a broken-winded horse and my hands hurt abominably. The saleroom string was coarse, hairy and abrasive and already it threatened to take the skin off my fingers.

Anyway, I thought, the worst was over. The tram stop was just at the end of the block there. I joined the queue and when the tram arrived, shuffled forward with the others. I had one foot on the step when a large hand was thrust before my eyes.

'Just a minute, brother, just a minute! Where d'you think you're goin'?' The face under the conductor's hat was the meaty, heavy jowled, pop-eyed kind which seems to take a mournful pleasure in imparting bad news.

'You're not bringin' that bloody lot on 'ere, brother, I'll tell tha now!'

I looked up at him in dismay. 'But ... it's just a few books ...'

'Few books! You want a bloody delivery van for that lot. You're not usin' my tram – passengers couldn't stir inside!' His mouth turned down aggressively.

'Oh but really,' I said with a ghastly attempt at an ingratiating smile, 'I'm just going as far as ...'

'You're not goin' anywhere in 'ere, brother! Ah've no time to argue – move your foot, ah'm off!'

The bell ding-dinged and the tram began to move. As I hopped off backwards one of the strings broke again.

After I had got myself sorted out I surveyed my situation and it appeared fairly desperate. My car must be over a mile away, mostly uphill, and I would defy the most stalwart Nepalese Sherpa to transport these books that far. I could of course just abandon the things; lean them against this wall and take to my heels ... But no, that would be anti-social and anyway they were beautiful. If only I could get them home all would be well.

Another tram rumbled up to the stop and again I hefted my

burden and joined the in-going passengers, hoping nobody would notice.

It was a female voice this time.

'Sorry, you can't come on, luv.' She was middle-aged, motherly and her plump figure bulged her uniform tightly.

'We don't 'ave delivery men on our trams. It's against t'rules.'

I repressed a scream. 'But I'm not a . . . these are my own books. I've just bought them.'

'Bought 'em?' Her eyebrows went up as she stared at the dusty columns.

'Yes . . . and I've got to get them home somehow.'

'Well somebody'll tek 'em home for you luv. Hasta got far to go?'

'Darrowby.'

'Eee, by gum, that's a long way. Right out in t'country.' She peered into the tram's interior. 'But there isn't no room in there, luv.'

The passengers had all filed in and I was left alone standing between my twin edifices; and the conductress must have seen a desperate light in my eyes because she made a sudden gesture.

'Come on then, luv! You stand out 'ere on the platform wi' me. I'm not supposed to, but ah can't see you stuck there.'

I didn't know whether to kiss her or burst into tears. In the end I did neither but stacked the books in a corner of the platform and stood swaying over them till we arrived at the park where I had left my car.

The relief at my deliverance was such that I laughed off the few extra contretemps on my way to the car. There were in fact several more spills before I had the books tucked away on the back seat but when I finally drove away I felt like singing.

It was when I was threading my way through the traffic that I began to rejoice that I lived in the country, because the car was filled with an acrid reek which I thought could only come from the conglomeration of petrol fumes and industrial smoke. But even when the city had been left behind and I was climbing into the swelling green of the Pennines the aroma was still with me.

I wound down the window and gulped greedily as the sweet grassy air flowed in but when I closed it the strange pungency returned immediately. I stopped, leaned over and sniffed at the region of the back seat. And there was no doubt about it; it was the books.

Ah well, they must have been kept in a damp place or something like that. I was sure it would soon pass off. But in the meantime it certainly was powerful; it nearly made my eyes water.

I had never really noticed the long climb to our eyrie on top of Skeldale House but it was different today. I suppose my arms and shoulders were finally beginning to feel the strain and that string, bristly but fragile, was digging into my hands harder than ever, but it was true that every step was an effort and when I at last gained the top landing I almost collapsed against the door of our bed-sitter.

When, perspiring and dishevelled, I entered, Helen was on her knees, dusting the hearth. She looked up at me expectantly.

'Any luck, Jim?'

'Yes, I think so,' I replied with a trace of smugness. 'I think I got a bargain.'

Helen rose and looked at me eagerly. 'Really?'

'Yes.' I decided to play my trump card. 'I only had to spend three shillings!'

'Three shillings! What ... where ...?'

'Wait there a minute.' I went out to the landing and put my hand under those strings. This, thank heaven, would be the last time I would have to do this. A lunge and a heave and I had my prizes through the doorway and displayed for my wife's inspection.

She stared at the two piles. 'What have you got there?'

'*The Geography of the World in Twenty Four Volumes,*' I replied triumphantly.

'The Geography of the ... and is that all?'

'Yes, couldn't manage anything else, I'm afraid. But look – aren't they magnificent books!'

My wife's level gaze had something of disbelief, a little of wonder. For a moment one corner of her mouth turned up then she coughed and became suddenly brisk.

'Ah well, we'll have to see about getting some shelves for them. Anyway, leave them there for now.' She went over and kneeled again by the hearth. But after a minute or two she paused in her dusting.

'Can you smell anything funny?'

'Well, er . . . I think it's the books, Helen. They're just a bit musty . . . I don't think it'll last long.'

But the peculiar exhalation was very pervasive and it was redolent of extreme age. Very soon the atmosphere in our room was that of a freshly opened mausoleum.

I could see Helen didn't want to hurt my feelings but she kept darting looks of growing alarm at my purchases. I decided to say it for her.

'Maybe I'd better take them downstairs just for now.'

She nodded gratefully.

The descent was torture, made worse by the fact that I had thought I was finished with such things. I finally staggered into the office and parked the books behind the desk. I was panting and rubbing my hands when Siegfried came in.

'Ah, James, had a nice run through to Leeds?'

'Yes, they said at the lab that they'd give us a ring about those sheep as soon as they've cultured the organisms.'

'Splendid!' My colleague opened the door of the cupboard and put some forms inside then he paused and began to sniff the air.

'James, there's a bloody awful stink in here.'

I cleared my throat. 'Well yes, Siegfried, I bought a few books while I was in Leeds. They seem a little damp.' I pointed behind the desk.

Siegfried's eyes widened as he looked at the twin edifices. 'What the devil are they?'

I hesitated. '*The Geography of the World in Twenty Four Volumes.*'

He didn't say anything but looked from me to the books and back again. And he kept sniffing. There was no doubt that only his innate good manners were preventing him from telling me to get the damn things out of here.

'I'll find a place for them,' I said, and with a great weariness pushed my hands yet again under the strings. My mind was in a ferment as I shuffled along the passage. What in heaven's name was I going to do with them? But as I passed the cellar door on my right it seemed to provide the answer.

There were great vaulted chambers beneath Skeldale House, a proper wine cellar in the grand days. The man who went down there to read the gas meter always described them as 'The Cattycombs' and as I descended into the murky, dank-smelling depths I thought sadly that it was a fitting resting place for my books. We kept only coal and wood down here now and from the muffled thuds I judged that Tristan was chopping logs.

He was a great log chopper and when I rounded the corner he was whirling his axe expertly round his head. He stopped when he saw me with my burden and asked the inevitable question.

I answered for, I hoped, the last time. '*The Geography of the World in Twenty Four Volumes.*' And I followed with a blow by blow account of my story.

As he listened he opened one tome after another, sniffed at it and replaced it hurriedly. And he didn't have to tell me, I knew already. My cherished books were down here to stay.

But the compassion which has always been and still is uppermost among the many facets of Tristan's character came to the fore now.

'Tell you what, Jim,' he said. 'We can put them in there.' He pointed to a dusty wine bin just visible in the dim light which filtered through the iron grating at the top of the coal chute which led from the street.

'It's just like a proper book shelf.'

He began to lift the volumes into the bin and when he had arranged them in a long row he ran his finger along the faded opulence of the bindings.

'There now, they look a treat in there, Jim.' He paused and rubbed his chin. 'Now all you want is somewhere to sit. Let's see now ... ah, yes!' He retreated into the gloom and reappeared with an armful of the biggest logs. He made a few more journeys and in no time had rigged up a seat for me within arm's reach of the books.

'That'll do fine,' he said with deep satisfaction. 'You can come down here and have a read whenever you feel like it.'

And that is how it turned out. The books never came up those steps again but quite frequently when I had a few minutes to spare and wanted to improve my mind I went down and sat on Tristan's seat in the twilight under the grating and renewed my acquaintance with *The Geography of the World in Twenty Four Volumes*.

16

I was sitting at the desk in the office at Skeldale House, writing up tuberculin testing forms when a young woman tapped on the door and walked in.

'I think I'm pregnant,' she murmured shyly.

I looked up at her in some surprise. It was an unusual opening to a conversation and I didn't quite know how to reply. She was about my own age and her demure attractiveness and rather prim style of dress didn't seem to belong to one so outspoken.

A furtive glance at her left hand did not help. She was wearing gloves so I was unable to use the presence or absence of a wedding ring to say either 'Congratulations' or 'Bad luck'.

'Really?' I replied lamely and followed it up with what I hoped was a non-committal smile.

'Yes, I think so.' She looked down and smoothed a finger along the strap of her handbag. Then she faced me again with an expectant expression as though she was waiting for me to make a move or say something helpful.

I dredged my mind desperately. There ought to be a fitting rejoinder somewhere but at the moment it escaped me. The silence was becoming embarrassing when the girl spoke again.

'Will you be able to examine me tonight?'

My face must have registered extreme emotion because she continued hastily.

'If it isn't suitable . . . I could come tomorrow night, doctor.'

Suddenly all was clear and I began to relax. The fact that our surgery was right next door to that of the local medicos gave rise to various contretemps but this was something new. Usually it was somebody wandering aimlessly along the passage, 'Looking for t'doctor', and they invariably left hastily when they discovered our identity. People often say to me, 'Vets must know just as much as doctors' but when it comes to the crunch they are never very keen to let me treat them.

There were notable exceptions to this rule among the older breed of farmers. Quite a few of these tough old men came to consult us about their rheumatism or their indigestion because 'them fellers next door never do me any bloody good.'

But usually it was just the accidental visitor and the doctors in their turn occasionally had their surgery hour enlivened by a lady marching in with a shaggy creature on a lead and asking them to squeeze out its anal glands.

I stood up and gave the girl a reassuring smile, while my mind ticked over busily. It seemed to me that in her delicate condition the sudden revelation that she was in the presence of a veterinary surgeon might have disastrous effects. So I took her gently by the arm, steered her from the room and along the passage to the front door. Still preserving a discreet silence I escorted her over the few yards of pavement to where our medical colleagues' plates hung by their entrance. I opened the door, led her inside, ushered her into the waiting room among the patient rows of country folk sitting there, gave her a final smile and nod, and fled.

There was another night when Tristan and I were tidying up after a cat spay. The sound of heavy boots echoed on the passage tiles then the door burst open and a stocky man in a cloth cap and collarless shirt strode in.

'I'm not goin' to be waitin' along there!' he said belligerently in the rich tones of Erin.

'Is that so?' I replied.

'Yiss, it is so. I haven't the time to be sittin' waitin'!'

'I see. Well what can we do for you?'

He grabbed a chair, pulled it up to the table, sat down, leaned his elbow on the freshly washed surface and looked up at me with a truculent eye.

'It's me ear!' He cocked the offending organ in my direction.

I realised he was one of the many Irish labourers who came to the district every year to help with the turnip hoeing. I could understand his entering the wrong door but was surprised at his aggressiveness; most of his compatriots were noted for their charm.

I was about to redirect him when Tristan, loth as always to pass up the slightest chance of a giggle, broke in.

'Your ear, eh?' he murmured sympathetically. 'Is it very painful?'

'Oh aye, it hurts bad. I think I've got a little bile startin' in there.'

Tristan tut-tutted. 'Too bad, too bad, let's have a look at it.' He moved over to the instrument cupboard and produced the auroscope which we used for examining dogs with ear canker. Taking it from its case he switched on the light and bent over the man.

'Just bend your head over a little, will you? Fine, fine.' He sounded very professional.

He inserted the auroscope and peered into the depths of the ear. 'Hmm . . . hmm . . . yes, yes, I see. Oh that's rather nasty.' At last he nodded gently. 'You are quite right. You have a little infected spot in there.'

'That's what I thought,' the man grunted. 'What are you going to do, then?'

Tristan rested his chin on his hands for a moment.

'I really think I ought to give you an injection. It would be the quickest way of clearing the thing up.' He spoke seriously but confidently with the hint of a grave smile at the corner of his lips. Like me he was wearing a white coat and would have passed without a quibble as a Harley Street specialist.

The man seemed similarly impressed. He squared his shoulders and nodded. 'Right then, let's be havin' it. You ought to know.'

As I watched wonderingly Tristan laid our white enamel tray on the table and on it he deposited a roll of cotton wool, a bottle of iodine and a row of enormous needles. They were the big, wide-bored needles for running calcium under a cow's skin and lying there they looked like items from a plumber's kit.

Next he rummaged in a cupboard for some time then emerged bearing the only 100 c.c. syringe in the practice. This was very rarely used – occasionally for giving sodium iodide injections to bullocks – and it was a fearsome object. Unlike its modern plastic counterparts it was made of glass and with its massive mounting of stainless steel and great metal plunger it looked much bigger.

The Irishman had been shifting uneasily in his seat as Tristan set out his stall but as the syringe clattered down on the enamel his eyes widened and he swallowed a couple of times.

My colleague, however, was wonderfully composed. He whistled softly as he fitted one of the huge needles to the nozzle of the syringe, then hummed a light tune while he hoisted a jar of acrivlavine solution on to the table. Carefully, almost lovingly, he drew up the full 100 c.c.'s then stood with the syringe poised against the light, giving off iridescent gleams as he rocked it gently to and fro.

The man had lost a lot of his bluster. His mouth hung slightly open.

'Just a minute,' he said a trifle breathlessly. 'Phwhaat doctors are you ?'

'I beg your pardon,' enquired Tristan, still juggling with his dreadful instrument.

'Phwhaat's your names ? Phwhaat do you call you doctors ?'

Tristan gave a light laugh. 'Oh we're not doctors. We're vets.'

'Vits!' the chair grated on the floor as the man pushed back from the table.

'Yes, that's right,' Tristan said innocently, advancing with the loaded syringe. 'But you needn't worry. I assure you . . .'

I don't think I have ever seen anybody leave a room as quickly as that man. His chair overturned, there was a scurry, a scraping of hobnails, the clattering of fleeing feet in the passage then the banging of the outside door.

He was gone, never to return . . .

I don't think there is much doubt that we held an earthy fascination for our medical colleagues. They were constantly drifting in to watch us at work, particularly my own doctor, Harry Allinson, whose bald head often hovered over me as I operated on the small animals.

'I've got to hand it to you boys,' he used to say. 'When we come up against a surgical case we write a note to the hospital but you just switch on the steriliser.'

He was interested, too, in our work with the microscope. It intrigued him that we should spend so much time peering down at skin scrapings for mange, blood films for anthrax milk and sputum smears for tuberculosis.

'Sometimes I think you are a really scientific chap, Jim,' he would laugh. 'Then I see you with your instruments.'

He was referring to the occasions when he met me coming out of the surgery in the morning carrying my kit for the round; the grisly docking knives, firing tools, tooth forceps and dehorning shears which are now mercifully consigned to the museum. He would lift them from my arms and examine them wonderingly. 'You put the horse's tail in there, do you? And you bring the blade down like this . . . bang . . . just like a guillotine . . . my God!'

I felt the same way myself.

Harry Allinson's towering, wide-shouldered frame was part of the scenery of Darrowby. He was a Scot, like so many of the doctors in Yorkshire, a great athlete in his youth, a scratch golfer and an ebullient personality. One of his main characteristics was sheer noisiness and it was his habit to march into his patients' homes shouting and banging about. He was to deliver both my children and years later when one or the other was ill I have heard him come hollering into the house . . . 'Anybody in? Who's there? Come on, let's be having you!' And it was wonderful how the little measles-ridden form revived and began to shout back at him.

It was rewarding, too, to discover the gentleness and understanding behind the uproar. Those qualities were always there when people needed them.

Although he saw so much of my own work I was unable, naturally enough, to see him in action apart from when he was attending my own family. There was one time, however, when I did have a peep behind the curtain.

I was called to see a lame cart horse and as I walked on to the farm I was surprised to see the vast form of Gobber Newhouse almost obscuring the view. The entire twenty stones of him was leaning on a shovel and he appeared to be part of a gang of building workers putting up a new barn.

'Nah then, Herriot,' he said affably, 'what've ye been killin' this mornin'?' He followed this typical sally with a throaty chuckle and looked round at his colleagues for applause.

I gave him a nod and passed by. Fortunately I didn't often see Gobber but when I did he always addressed me as 'Herriot' and he invariably got in some little dig. And incidentally this was the first time I had ever observed him going through the motions of work; the Labour Exchange must have put some pressure on him because normally his life consisted of drinking, gambling, fighting and knocking his long-suffering little wife about.

I spent some time with the horse's hind foot resting on my knee as I pared away at the sole. But there was no sign of pus and the only abnormality was a smelly disintegration of the horn around the frog.

'He's got thrush,' I said to the farmer. 'This doesn't often make them lame but he has shed quite a lot of horn and some of the sensitive tissues are exposed. I'll leave you some lotion for him.'

I was walking back to get the bottle from the car when I saw there was some kind of commotion among the builder's men. They were standing in a group around Gobber who was seated on an upturned milk pail. He had his boot off and was anxiously examining his foot.

The foreman called over to me. 'Are you going straight back to Darrowby, Mr Herriot?'

'Yes, I am.'

'Well maybe you wouldn't mind givin' this feller a lift. He's stood on a nail – went clean through his boot. Could you take him to a doctor?'

'Yes, of course.' I went over and viewed the fat man whose mates seemed to be enjoying the situation.

'Here's the vet come to see ye, Gobber,' one of them cried. 'He'll soon fix you up. He's been doctorin' t'oss's foot, now he can do yours. Will we haud 'im down for ye, Mr Herriot?'

Another peered gloomily at the punctured wound on the foot. 'By Gaw, this is a 'ell of a farm for lockjaw, Gobber. Ah'm afraid ye'll die a 'orrible death.'

The big man was not amused. His face was a tragic mask and the effort of hauling his foot into view above his enormous belly made him shake uncontrollably.

I opened the car door and, supported by a man on either side, he limped with many facial contortions across the farmyard. At first I thought we'd never be able to get him into the little vehicle and he groaned piteously as we pushed, pulled and finally wedged him into the passenger seat.

As we headed along the road to Darrowby he cleared his throat nervously.

'Mr Herriot,' he said. It was the first time he had ever accorded me a 'Mister'. 'Is it true that where there's a lot of 'osses there's more lockjaw?'

'Yes, I should say so,' I replied.

He swallowed. 'There's allus been a lot of 'osses at that farm, hasn't there?'

'There has indeed.'

'And what . . .' He passed a hand across his forehead. 'What kind of . . . er . . . cuts gets lockjaw in them?'

I saw no reason to be merciful. 'Oh, deep punctured wounds like you have. Especially in the feet.'

'Oh bloody 'ell!' moaned Gobber. Like many bullies he was a big baby when his own hide was in danger.

Watching him sweating there I relented a little.

'Don't worry,' I said. 'The doctor will give you a little shot and you'll have nothing to worry about.'

The big man squirmed and wrung his hands. 'Ah but I don't like t'needle.'

'It's nothing, really,' I said, with only the slightest touch of sadism. 'Just a quick jab.'

'Oh bloody 'ell!'

At the surgery Harry Allinson gave us a cold look as we staggered in. He had attended a few of Mrs Newhouse's black eyes and he didn't approve of Gobber.

'Right, Jim,' he grunted. 'Leave him to me.'

I was about to go when Gobber caught at my sleeve.

'Stay with me, Mr Herriot!' he whimpered. The man was in a pitiable state of fright and I looked questioningly at the doctor.

Harry shrugged. 'OK, you can stay and hold his hand if that's what he wants.'

He produced a phial of tetanus antitoxin and a syringe.

'Drop your trousers and bend over, Newhouse,' he ordered curtly.

Gobber complied, exposing flaccid acres of the biggest backside, horses included, which I had ever seen.

'You know, Newhouse,' Harry said conversationally as he filled the syringe before the big man's terrified eyes. 'Your wife tells me you have no feelings.' He laughed gently. 'Yes, that's what she says . . . you have absolutely no feelings.'

He stepped quickly to the rear, rammed the needle deep into the quivering buttock, then, as a shrill howl shook the windows, he looked into Gobber's face with a wolfish grin.

'But you bloody well felt that, didn't you!'

17

You often see dogs running along a road but there was something about this one which made me slow down and take a second look.

It was a small brown animal and it was approaching on the other side; and it wasn't just ambling by the grass verge but galloping all out on its short legs, head extended forward as though in desperate pursuit of something unseen beyond the long empty curve of tarmac ahead. As the dog passed I had a brief glimpse of two staring eyes and a lolling tongue, then he was gone.

My car stalled and lurched to a halt but I sat unheeding, still gazing into the mirror at the small form receding rapidly until it was almost invisible against the browns and greens of the surrounding moor. As I switched on the engine I had difficulty in dragging my thoughts back to the job in hand; because I had seen something chilling there, a momentary but vivid impression of frantic effort, despair, blind terror. And driving away, the image stayed with me. Where had that dog come from? There were no roadside farms on this high, lonely by-way, not a parked car anywhere. And in any case he wasn't just casually going somewhere; there was a frenzied urgency in his every movement.

It was no good, I had to find out. I backed off the unfenced road among the sparse tufts of heather and turned back in the direction I had come. I had to drive a surprisingly long way before I saw the little animal, still beating his solitary way, and at the sound of the approaching car he halted, stared for a moment then trotted on again. But his labouring limbs told me he was near exhaustion and I pulled up twenty yards ahead of him, got out and waited.

He made no protest as I knelt on the roadside turf and caught him gently as he came up to me. He was a Border terrier and after another quick glance at the car his eyes took on their terrified light as he looked again at the empty road ahead.

He wasn't wearing a collar but there was a ring of flattened hair on his neck as though one had recently been removed. I opened his mouth and looked at his teeth; he wasn't very old – probably around two or three. There were rolls of fat along his ribs so he hadn't been starved. I was examining his skin when suddenly the wide panting mouth closed and the whole body stiffened as another car approached. For a moment he stared at it with fierce hope but when the vehicle flashed by he sagged and began to pant again.

So that was it. He had been dumped. Some time ago the humans he had loved and trusted had opened their car door, hurled him out into an unknown world and driven merrily away. I began to feel sick – physically sick – and a murderous rage flowed through me. Had they laughed, I wondered, these people, at the idea of the bewildered little creature toiling vainly behind them?

I passed my hand over the rough hairs of the head. I could forgive anybody for robbing a bank but never for this. 'Come on, fella,' I said, lifting him gently, 'you're coming home with me.'

Sam was used to strange dogs in the car and he sniffed incuriously at the newcomer. The terrier huddled on the passenger seat trembling violently and I kept my hand on him as I drove.

Back in our bed-sitter Helen pushed a bowl of meat and biscuit under his nose but the little animal showed no interest.

'How could anybody do this?' she murmured. 'And anyway, why? What reason could they have?'

I stroked the head again. 'Oh, you'd be surprised at some of the reasons. Sometimes they do it because a dog turns savage, but that can't be so in this case.' I had seen enough of dogs to interpret the warm friendly light behind the fear in those eyes. And the way the terrier had submitted unquestioningly as I had prised his mouth open, lifted him, handled him, all pointed to one thing; he was a docile little creature.

'Or sometimes,' I continued, 'they dump dogs just because

they're tired of them. They got them when they were charming puppies and have no interest in them when they grow up. Or maybe the licence is due to be paid – that's a good enough reason for some people to take a drive into the country and push their pets out into the unknown.'

I didn't say any more. There was quite a long list and why should I depress Helen with tales of the other times when I had seen it happen? People moving to another house where they couldn't keep a dog. A baby arriving and claiming all the attention and affection. And dogs were occasionally abandoned when a more glamorous pet superseded them.

I looked at the little terrier. This was the sort of thing which could have happened to him. A big dashing Alsatian, an eye-catching Saluki – anything like that would take over effortlessly from a rather roly-poly Border terrier with some people. I had seen it in the past. The little fellow was definitely running to fat despite his comparative youth; in fact when he had been running back there his legs had splayed out from his shoulders. That was another clue; it was possible he had spent most of his time indoors without exercise.

Anyway I was only guessing. I rang the police. No reports of a lost dog in the district. I hadn't really expected any.

During the evening we did our best to comfort the terrier but he lay trembling, his head on his paws, his eyes closed. The only time he showed interest was when a car passed along the street outside, then he would raise his head and listen, ears pricked, for a few seconds till the sound died away. Helen hoisted him on to her lap and held him there for over an hour, but he was too deeply sunk in his misery to respond to her caresses and soft words.

I finally decided it would be the best thing to sedate him and gave him a shot of morphine. When we went to bed he was stretched out sound asleep in Sam's basket with Sam himself curled up philosophically on the rug by his side.

Next morning he was still unhappy but sufficiently recovered to look around him and take stock. When I went up and spoke to him he rolled over on his back, not playfully but almost automatically as though it was a normal mannerism. I bent and rubbed his chest while he looked up at me non-committally. I liked dogs which rolled over like this; they were usually good-natured and it was a gesture of trust.

'That's better, old lad,' I said. 'Come on, cheer up!'

For a moment his mouth opened wide. He had a comical little monkey face and briefly it seemed to be split in two by a huge grin, making him look extraordinarily attractive.

Helen spoke over my shoulder. 'He's a lovely little dog, Jim! He's so appealing – I could get really fond of him.'

Yes, that was the trouble. So could I. I could get too fond of all the unwanted animals which passed through our hands; not just the abandoned ones but the dogs which came in for eutha-nasia with the traumatic addendum 'unless you can find him a home'. That put the pressure on me. Putting an animal to sleep when he was incurably ill, in pain, or so old that life had lost its savour was something I could tolerate. In fact often it seemed as though I were doing the suffering creature a favour. But when a young, healthy, charming animal was involved then it was a harrowing business.

What does a vet do in these circumstances. Refuse and send the owners away with the lurking knowledge that the man might go round to the chemist and buy a dose of poison? That was far worse than our humane, painless barbiturate. One thing a vet can't do is take in all those animals himself. If I had given way to all my impulses I would have accumulated a positive menagerie by now.

It was a hell of a problem which had always troubled me and now I had a soft hearted wife which made the pull twice as strong.

I turned to her now and voiced my thoughts.

'Helen, we can't keep him, you know. One dog in a bed-sitter is enough.' I didn't add that we ourselves probably would not be in the bed-sitter much longer; that was another thing I didn't want to bring up.

She nodded. 'I suppose so. But I have the feeling that this is one of the sweetest little dogs I've seen for a long time. When

124

he gets over his fear, I mean. What on earth can we do with him?'

'Well, he's a stray.' I bent again and rubbed the rough hair over the chest. 'So he should really go to the kennels at the police station. But if he isn't claimed in ten days we are back where we started.' I put my hand under the terrier's body and lifted him, limp and unresisting, into the crook of my arm. He liked people, this one; liked and trusted them. 'I could ask around the practice, of course, but nobody seems to want a dog when there's one going spare.' I thought for a moment or two. 'Maybe an advert in the local paper.'

'Wait a minute,' Helen said. 'Talking about the paper – didn't I read something about an animal shelter last week?'

I looked at her uncomprehendingly then I remembered.

'That's right. Sister Rose from the Topley Banks hospital. They were interviewing her about the stray animals she had taken in. It would be worth a try.' I replaced the terrier in Sam's basket. 'We'll keep this little chap today and I'll ring Sister Rose when I finish work tonight.'

At teatime I could see that things were getting out of hand. When I came in the little dog was on Helen's knee and it looked as though he had been there for a long time. She was stroking his head and looking definitely broody.

Not only that, but as I looked down at him I could feel myself weakening. Little phrases were creeping unbidden into my mind . . . 'I wonder if we could find room for him . . .' . . . 'Not much extra trouble . . .' . . . 'Perhaps if we . . .'

I had to act quickly or I was sunk. Reaching for the phone I dialled the hospital number. They soon found Sister Rose and I listened to a cheerful, businesslike voice. She didn't seem to find anything unusual in the situation and the matter-of-fact way she asked questions about the terrier's age, appearance, temperament etc. gave the impression that she had seen a lot of unwanted animals through her hands.

I could hear the firm pencilling sounds as she took notes then, 'Well now that sounds fine. He's the sort we can usually find a home for. When can you bring him along?'

125

'Now,' I replied.

The misty look in Helen's eyes as I marched out with the dog under my arm told me I was only just in time. And as I drove along the road I couldn't put away the thought that if things had been different – the future settled and a proper home – this little brown creature rolling on his back on the passenger seat with his wide mouth half open and the friendly eyes fixed questioningly on mine would never have got away from me. Only when the occasional car flashed by did he spring upright and look from the window with the old despairing expression. Would he ever forget?

Sister Louisa Rose was a rather handsome woman in her late forties with the sort of healthy smiling face I had imagined at the other end of the phone. She reached out and took the terrier from me with the eager gesture of the animal lover.

'Oh, he looks rather a dear, doesn't he?' she murmured.

Behind her house, a modern bungalow in the open country near the hospital, she led me to a row of kennels with outside runs. Some of them housed single dogs but there was one large one with an assortment of mixed breeds playing happily together on the grass.

'I think we'll put him in here,' she said. 'It'll cheer him up quicker than anything and I'm sure he'll mix in well.' She opened a door in the wire netting surround and pushed the little animal in. The other dogs surrounded him and there was the usual ceremonious sniffing and leg-cocking.

Sister Rose cupped her chin with her hand and looked down thoughtfully through the wire. 'A name, we must have a name ... let me see ... no ... no ... yes ... Pip! We'll call him Pip!'

She looked at me with raised eyebrows and I nodded vigorously. 'Yes, definitely – just right. He looks like a Pip.'

She smiled impishly. 'I think so, too, but I've had a lot of practice, you know. I've become rather good at it.'

'I'll bet you have. I suppose you've named all this lot?'

'Of course.' She began to point them out one by one. 'There's Bingo – he was a badly neglected puppy. And Fergus – just lost. That bigger retriever is Griff – he was the survivor of a car crash

126

where his owners were killed. And Tessa, badly injured when she was thrown from a fast-moving vehicle. Behind her over there is Sally Anne who really started me in the business of Animal Sheltering. She was found heavily pregnant with her paws bleeding so she must have run for many miles. I took her in and managed to find homes for all her puppies and she's still here. Placing those pups got me into contact with a lot of pet owners and before I knew what was happening everybody had the idea that I regularly took in stray animals. So I started and you can see the result. I shall have to expand these premises soon.'

Pip didn't look so lonely now and after the preliminary courtesies he joined a group watching interestedly a fierce tug-of-war on a stick between a Collie and a crossed Labrador.

I laughed. 'You know I had no idea you had all these dogs. How long do you keep them?'

'Till I can find a home for them. Some are only here a day, others stay for weeks or months. And there are one or two like Sally Anne who seem to be permanent boarders now.'

'But how on earth do you feed them all? It must be an expensive business.'

She nodded and smiled. 'Oh I run little dog shows, coffee mornings, raffles, jumble sales, anything, but whatever my efforts I'm afraid the strays keep munching their way into the red. But I manage.'

She managed, I guessed, by dipping deeply into her own pocket. Around me the abandoned and rejected dogs barked and ran around happily. I had often thought when I encountered cruelty and neglect that there was a whole army of people who did these unspeakable things, a great unheeding horde who never spared a thought for the feelings of the helpless creatures who depended on them. It was frightening in a way, but thank heavens there was another army ranged on the other side, an army who fought for the animals with everything they had – with their energy, their time, their money.

I looked at Sister Rose, at the steady eyes in the clear-skinned, scrubbed, nurse's face. I would have thought her profession of dedication to the human race would have filled her life utterly with no room for anything else, but it was not so.

'Well, I'm very grateful to you, Sister,' I said. 'I hope somebody will take Pip off your hands soon and if there's anything else I can do, please let me know.'

She smiled. 'Oh don't worry, I have a feeling this little chap won't be here very long.'

Before leaving I leaned on the wire and took another look at the Border terrier. He seemed to be settling all right but every now and then he stopped and looked up at me with those questioning eyes which pulled so hard. I had the nasty feeling that I, too, was letting him down. His owners, then me, then Sister Rose, all in a couple of days . . . I hoped it would work out for him.

18

I found it difficult to get that dog out of my mind and I lasted only a week before dropping in at the Animal Shelter. Sister Rose in an old mackintosh and wellingtons was filling the feeding bowls in one of the kennels.

'You've come about Pip, I expect,' she said, putting down her bucket. 'Well he went yesterday. I thought I'd have no trouble. A very nice couple called round. They wanted to give a home to a stray and they picked him out straight away.' She pushed the hair back from her forehead. 'In fact I've had a good week. I've found excellent homes for Griff and Fergus too.'

'Fine, fine. That's great.' I paused for a moment. 'I was wondering . . . er . . . about Pip. Has he gone out of the district ?'

'Oh, no, he's right here in Darrowby. The people are called Plenderleith – he's a retired civil servant, quite high up I believe and he gave a generous donation to the centre though I didn't expect one. They've bought one of those nice little houses on the Houlton Road and there's a lovely garden for Pip to play. I gave them your name, by the way, so no doubt they'll be coming round to see you.'

A wave of totally irrational pleasure swept over me.

'Ah well, I'm glad to hear that. I'll be able to see how he's getting on.'

I didn't have long to wait. It was less than a week later that I opened the waiting-room door and saw an elderly couple sitting there with Pip on the end of a very new lead. He adopted his usual gambit of rolling on to his back as soon as he saw me, but this time there was no helpless appeal in his expression but sheer joyous abandon with the comical little face split across by a wide panting grin. As I went through the ritual of chest rubbing I noticed he was wearing a new collar, too; expensive looking, with a shining medallion bearing his name, address and tele-phone number. I lifted him and we all went through to the consulting room.

'Well now, what's the trouble?' I asked.

'No trouble, really,' the man replied. He was plump, and the pink face, grave eyes and immaculate dark suit accorded per-fectly with my idea of a top civil servant.

'I have recently acquired this small animal and should be grateful for your advice about him. By the way, my name is Plenderleith and may I introduce my wife.'

Mrs Plenderleith was plump too, but it was a giggly plump-ness. She didn't look such a solid citizen as her husband.

'Firstly,' he continued, 'I should like you to give him a thorough check-up.'

I had already done this, but went through it again, though Pip made things difficult by rolling over every time I got the stethoscope on his chest. And as I took his temperature I noticed that Mr Plenderleith ran his hand repeatedly over the brown hair of the back while his wife, looking over his shoulder, made encouraging noises and nodded reassuringly at the little dog.

'Absolutely sound in wind and limb,' I pronounced as I finished.

'Splendid,' the man said. 'Er . . . there was this little brown mark on his abdomen . . .' A touch of anxiety showed in his eyes.

'Just a patch of pigment. Nothing, I assure you.'

'Ah yes, good, good.' Mr Plenderleith cleared his throat. 'I have to confess, Mr Herriot, that my wife and I have never owned an animal before. Now I believe in doing things thoroughly, so in order to give him proper care and attention I have decided to study the matter. With this in view I have purchased some books on the subject.' He produced some shiny volumes from under his arm. *Care of the Dog*, *The Dog in Sickness and Health*, and finally *The Border Terrier*.

'Good idea,' I replied. Normally I would have shied away from this imposing battery but in this case I liked the way things were going. I had the growing conviction that Pip was on a good wicket here.

'I have already gleaned a considerable amount from my reading,' Mr Plenderleith went on, 'and I believe it is desirable that he be inoculated against distemper. As you know, he is a stray so there is no means of ascertaining whether or not this has been done.'

I nodded. 'Quite right. In fact I was going to suggest that.' I produced a phial of the vaccine and began to fill a syringe.

Pip was much less concerned than his owners as I gently injected the contents under his skin. Mr Plenderleith, his face rigid with apprehension, kept patting the dog's head while his wife at the other end stroked the hind limbs and adjured her pet to be brave.

After I had put the syringe away, Mr Plenderleith, visibly relieved, recommenced his investigations. 'Let me see now.' He put on his spectacles, produced a gold pencil and snapped open a leather bound pad where I could see a long list of neatly written notes. 'I have one or two queries here.'

And he had indeed. He grilled me at length on feeding, housing, exercise, the relative values of wicker dog baskets and metal frame beds, the salient features of the common ailments, often referring to his shiny books. 'I have a note here concerning page 143, line 9. It says . . .'

I answered him patiently, leaning across the table. I had a waiting list of farm visits including several fairly urgent jobs but I listened with growing contentment. I had hoped for concerned and responsible persons to take this little animal over and these people were right out of the blueprint.

When at length Mr Plenderleith had finished he put away his notebook and pencil and removed his spectacles with the firm precise movements which seemed part of him.

'One of the reasons I desired a dog, Mr Herriot,' he went on, 'was to provide myself with exercise. Don't you think that is a good idea?'

'It certainly is. One of the surest ways to keep fit is to own an active little animal like this. You simply *have* to take him out and just think of all the lovely grassy tracks over the hills around here. On Sunday afternoons when other people are lying asleep in their chairs under their newspapers you'll be out there striding the fells, rain, hail or snow.'

Mr Plenderleith squared his shoulders and his jaw jutted as though he already saw himself battling through a blizzard.

'And another thing,' his wife giggled, 'it'll take some of this off.' She thumped him irreverently on his bulging waistline.

'Now now, my dear,' he admonished her gravely, but I had seen the makings of a sheepish grin which completely belied his stuffed shirt image. Mr Plenderleith, I felt, was all right.

He put his books under his arm and reached out for the little dog. 'Come, Pip, we mustn't delay Mr Herriot any longer.' But his wife was too quick for him. She gathered the terrier into her arms and as we walked along the passage she held the rough face against her own.

Outside the surgery door I saw them installed in a spotless little family saloon and as they drove away Mr Plenderleith inclined his head gravely, his wife gave a gay wave, but Pip, his hind legs on her knee, feet on the dashboard, gazing eagerly through the windscreen was too busy and interested to look at me.

As they rounded the corner I had the impression of a little cycle coming to a happy end. And of course the main cog in the sequence of events had been Sister Rose. This was just one of the helpless creatures she had salvaged. Her Animal Shelter would grow and expand and daily she would work harder without gain to herself. There were other people like her all over the country, other Shelters; and I felt I had been given a privileged glimpse of that selfless army which battled ceaselessly and untiringly on the side of the great throng of dependent animals.

But right now I was concerned only with one thing. Pip had come home for good.

19

'Double Bezique!' Helen said, laying out the two queens of spades and the jacks of diamonds. And she looked across at me with a grin of triumph.

She had the right kind of mouth, wide and generous, for such a grin and there was no doubt she had cause for jubilation.

'Well that's torn it,' I grunted moodily. 'I've been wondering where those cards were and now I know. But why didn't you declare them separately?'

'It's better fun this way,' my wife replied with a callous laugh. 'I wanted to see your face when I put them all out at once.'

'OK, OK,' I said. 'Gloat all you want. I didn't realise I had married a sadist.'

With a sinking heart I saw her move her little peg five hundred points up the board. It was a body blow and one from which I knew I would never recover. She had already won two games tonight – I was being thrashed.

Still, there were compensations. There was a subdued excitement in just sitting there by our fireside on a black winter's night like this and listening to the wind buffeting the tall old house. I think it was the nearness of the wild that made the coals burn brighter and the room seem cosier, the awareness of the towering bare hills close by and the night wind shrieking over the high tops and over the vast white emptiness of the moors where it was cold, cold, and a man could quite easily lose himself and die.

I dealt the next hand and looked with disgust at the rubbish I had given myself. I stole a glance at Helen. The faintest trace of smugness showed in her face as she viewed her hand. This wasn't going to be my night.

We played a lot of Bezique on those dark evenings. There wasn't much to do in Darrowby but boredom was never a problem. At the beginning, in the summer days, we walked every day along the grassy tracks in the hills which make Yorkshire the finest walking country in England. We started to cultivate a piece of the long garden behind the house for our own use and I discovered an undreamed-of fascination in peas and broad beans. We picked mushrooms which may not sound very exciting but I have warm memories of the two of us wandering around sunlit fields with carrier bags and stopping now and then to look at the beauty nearby. In those days before the old permanent pastures were ploughed up and artificial fertilisers were scarcely used mushrooms grew abundantly; and they were marvellous to eat. There was tennis, too, and at weekends Helen came with me on my rounds.

But when the winter closed in Bezique was the thing. I studied my cards again and listened to the wind. It made a soft whistling noise down in the tiled passage far below. It was always as cold as the street in that passage and not much warmer in the graceful sitting room where the wind would tug at the heavy curtains over the french windows and perhaps send fugitive gusts up the stairs to Siegfried's and Tristan's rooms and then up to us on the top.

And the wind would push its fingers up under the tiles into the two empty silent rooms which lay even higher than us. Rooms where the dust lay thick beneath their tiny windows and the wind would stir the cobwebs among the rafters and pull at the little bell hanging from the great coiled spring. I could hear the faint tinkling which in the days of the old house's glory would summon a little maidservant from her high nest.

But now the bell went unheeded in the empty darkness. There was nobody to answer it. The six servants who used to look after the Georgian elegance of Skeldale House were only a memory among the older folk of Darrowby and there was only Mrs Hall the housekeeper in her room at the end of the offshoot.

'Royal marriage,' I said stiffly, putting out the king and queen of trumps and advancing my peg a paltry forty points.

Helen nodded and I could see she was trying not to look condescending. She hadn't declared anything for some time now and I had a nasty feeling she was building up to something big. She bent over and poked the fire. There was too much coal on it because I had laid the fire this evening.

We had a system that whoever was first home did that job. We had to arrange something like this because Helen was a working girl now. There wasn't much to do in our two rooms and our finances were at a low ebb so she had taken a job as secretary to the local millers. The mill was on the roadside down by the river and passers-by could see the big mill wheel turning in the water and hear the great stones grinding the corn in the room upstairs with the opening on to the road where the lorries came to collect the loaded bags.

Helen's office was behind the mill shop, a floury, dusty, mealy place stacked tightly with sacks of cow cake, sheep nuts, hen pellets and drums of black treacle and when I slowed down outside I could often catch a glimpse of her red-sweatered back as she bent over her books.

Tonight I had been first home and Helen had come in as I was lighting my pile of sticks and coal. Girls used to wear things called 'pixie hoods' in those days and I can see her now in a blue pixie hood, her face flushed with the long climb up the stairs looking round that door at me busy with my chores.

But tonight my worst fears were being realised. My wife gave a long contented sigh and laid out one by one the dread ace, king, queen, jack and ten.

'Sequence,' she murmured in a matter of fact tone and moved her peg up another two hundred and fifty.

It wasn't a defeat, it was a massacre. It was obvious I hadn't long to live. But as I scanned the board anxiously the front door bell echoed along the passage downstairs.

Maybe I was going to be saved. I leapt to my feet and began the familiar descent.

A bulky figure loomed beyond the glass door at the end of the passage and as I turned the handle a waft of beer fumes blew in.

'Ah want a cleansing drink,' the figure said.

I opened the door wide. 'Come inside for a minute, it's a cold night.'

It was Reg Mallaby, a member of the large body of farmers who liked to drop in at the surgery on the way home after a night in the pub or the cinema, just to pick up some medicaments for the livestock.

We went into the office and he stood leaning on the desk, breathing heavily.

'A cleansing drink, eh?' I said. 'Right, I'll bring one through.'

Of course there was no such thing as a cleansing drink – there never has been – and when I first came to Darrowby and didn't know any better I used to waste a lot of time telling the farmers so. I went out of my way to explain as lucidly as I could that nothing you poured down a cow's throat could possibly influence the separation of the afterbirth and that they shouldn't throw their money away on something which was useless. The farmers listened with growing disbelief then left, offended, to purchase a cleansing drink at the chemist's shop.

I took a more practical view now and went through to the stock-room. There was quite a pile of the square packets there. They were wrapped in bright red paper with lettering in confident black capitals and we did a brisk trade in them at half a crown a time. We bought them by the gross from a wholesaler and though I never had them analysed I had a strong suspicion that they consisted of a pound of Epsom salts flavoured with aromatic powder.

'Here you are, Mr Mallaby,' I said. 'That's what you want, isn't it?'

'Aye, that's it, young man.' The farmer handled the packet almost lovingly. 'They're champion things, these, tha knows. Ah've never known 'em fail. Must have some wonderful stuff in 'em.'

He handed over his half crown then looked at me benevolently. 'I 'ope I haven't disturbed you, lad. Maybe you were doing summat important like?'

'No, that's quite all right, Mr Mallaby.' I looked at him with mingled surprise and gratitude. He was the first of the nocturnal callers who had shown any interest or concern. It had always been another symptom of the general opinion that vets have no private life. 'No, you needn't worry about that. I was just playing cards with my wife.'

The farmer nodded and a slow seraphic smile crept over his face. There was no doubt he had been indulging to the full. Then he narrowed his eyes suddenly.

'Is your Missus t'lass that works at t'mill?'

'Yes, that's right. She's in the office there.'

His face became very solemn. 'Aye well, I 'ave a complaint to make.'

'A complaint? What do you mean?'

I must have looked astonished because he held up a placatory hand.

'Now then, young man, she's a grand lass, I'm not sayin' nowt about that. But she sent me a wrong bill.'

'A wrong bill? In what way?'

'There was a mistake in it. She charged me for a lot o' things I never 'ad.'

'Well that's very strange. Are you absolutely sure?' I could easily imagine myself making clerical errors but in my experience Helen was a model of efficiency in that line.

'Aye, ah'm sure,' he replied. 'Haud on a minute and I'll show you. I 'ave it in my pocket here.'

He put his cleansing drink on the desk and began a laborious search of his pockets. He tracked down the offending account among a huge wad of envelopes which he extracted from inside his coat.

'There y'are, young man,' he said importantly. 'Just have a look at that.'

I studied the paper carefully. Opposite a date at the top there was an entry. 'Two bags pig meal' and underneath on dates when the order had obviously been repeated Helen had put dittos by writing 'do . . . do . . . do . . . do'.

'Well what's wrong with it, Mr Mallaby?'

The farmer pursed his lips. 'Ah'll tell ye. Ye see that about pig meal?'

I nodded.

'Well,' he went on, 'ah've had a few bags o' that, I'm not denyin' and I expect to pay for't. But . . .' and here he raised a portentous forefinger, 'there's one thing I'm certain of. Ah've never 'ad none o' them bloody doo-doo's.'

20

No vet likes to have his job made more difficult and as I worked inside the ewe I fought a rising tide of irritation.

'You know, Mr Kitson,' I said testily, 'you should have got me out sooner. How long have you been trying to lamb this ewe?'

The big man grunted and shrugged his shoulders. 'Oh, for a bit – not ower long.'

'Half an hour – an hour?'

'Nay, nay, nobbut a few minutes.' Mr Kitson regarded me gloomily along his pointed nose. It was his habitual expression; in fact I had never seen him smile and the idea of a laugh ever disturbing those pendulous cheeks was unthinkable.

I gritted my teeth and decided to say no more about it, but I knew it had taken more than a few minutes to cause the swelling of the vaginal wall, this sandpaper dryness of the little creatures inside. And it was a simple enough presentation – biggish twins, one anterior the other posterior, but of course as often happens the hind legs of one were laid alongside the head of the other giving the illusion that they belonged to the same lamb. I'd like to bet that Mr Kitson had been guddling for ages inside her with his big rough hands in a dogged attempt to bring that head and those legs out together.

If I had been there at the start it would have been the work of a few moments but instead here I was without an inch of space, trying to push things around with one finger instead of my full hand and getting nowhere.

Fortunately the present day farmer doesn't often play this trick on us. The usual thing I hear at a lambing is, 'Nay, I just had a quick feel and I knew it wasn't a job for me,' or something I heard from a farmer the other day, 'Two men at one ewe's no good,' and I think that says it very well.

But Mr Kitson was of the old school. He didn't believe in getting the vet out until every other avenue had been explored and when he did finally have to fall back on our services he was usually dissatisfied with the result.

'This is no good,' I said, withdrawing my hand and swilling it quickly in the bucket. 'I'll have to do something about this dryness.'

I walked the length of the old stable which had been converted into temporary lambing pens and lifted a tube of lubricating cream from the car boot. Coming in again I heard a faint sound from my left. The stable was dimly lit and an ancient door had been placed across the darkest corner to make a small enclosure. I looked inside and in the gloom could just discern a ewe lying on her chest, head outstretched. Her ribs rose and fell with the typical quick distressed respirations of a sheep in pain. Occasionally she moaned softly.

'What's the trouble here?' I asked.

Mr Kitson regarded me impassively from the other end of the building. 'She 'ad a roughish time lambin' yesterday.'

'How do you mean, roughish?'

'Well . . . a big single lamb wi' a leg back and I couldn't fetch it round.'

'So you just pulled it out as it was . . . with the leg back?'

'Aye, nowt else ah could do.'

I leaned over the door and lifted the ewe's tail, filthy with faeces and discharge. I winced as I saw the tumefied, discoloured vulva and perineum.

'She could do with a bit of attention, Mr Kitson.'

The farmer looked startled. 'Nay, nay, I don't want none o' that. It's over with her – there's nowt you can do.'

'You mean she's dying?'

'That's right.'

I put my hand on the sheep's head, feeling the coldness of the ears and lips. He could be right.

'Well have you rung Mallock to come and pick her up? She really should be put out of her pain as soon as possible.'

'Aye . . . ah'll do that.' Mr Kitson shuffled his feet and looked away.

I knew what the situation was. He was going to let the ewe 'take her chance'. The lambing season was always a rewarding and fulfilling time for me but this was the other side of the coin. It was a hectic time in the farming year, a sudden onslaught of extra work on top of the routine jobs and in some ways it overwhelmed the resources of farmers and vets alike. The flood of new life left a pathetic debris behind it; a flotsam and jetsam of broken creatures; ewes too old to stand a further pregnancy, some debilitated by diseases like liver fluke and toxaemia, others with infected arthritic joints and others who had just had a 'roughish time'. You were inclined to find them lying half forgotten in dark corners like the one in this stable. They had been left there to 'take their chance'.

I returned in silence to my original patient. My lubricating cream made a great difference and I was able to use more than one finger to explore. I had to make up my mind whether to repel the posterior or anterior presentation and since the head was well into the vagina I decided to bring out the anterior first.

With the farmer's help I raised the ewe's hindquarters till they were resting on a straw bale. I could work downhill now and gently pushed the two hind limbs away into the depths of the uterus. In the space which this left I was able to hook a finger round the fore limbs which were laid back along the ribs of the anterior lamb and bring them into the passage. I only needed another application of the cream and a few moments' careful traction and the lamb was delivered.

But it was all too late. The tiny creature was quite dead and the knell of disappointment sounded in me as it always did at the sight of the perfectly formed body which lacked only the spark of life.

Hurriedly I greased my arm again and felt inside for the re-pelled lamb. There was plenty of room now and I was able to loop my hand round the hocks and draw the lamb out without effort. This time I had little hope of life and my efforts were solely to relieve the ewe's discomfort but as the lamb came into the cold outside air I felt the convulsive jerk and wriggle of the woolly little form in my hands which told me all was well.

It was funny how often this happened; you got a dead lamb – sometimes even a decomposed one – with a live one lurking behind it. Anyway it was a bonus and with a surge of pleasure I wiped the mucus from its mouth and pushed it forward for its mother to lick. A further exploration of the uterus revealed nothing more and I got to my feet.

'Well she's come to no harm, and I think she'll be all right now,' I said. 'And could I have some fresh water, Mr Kitson, please?'

The big man wordlessly emptied the bucket on to the stable floor and went off towards the house. In the silence I could faintly hear the panting of the ewe in the far corner. I tried not to think of what lay in front of her. Soon I would drive off and see other cases, then I would have lunch and start my afternoon round while hidden in this cheerless place a helpless animal was gasping her life away. How long would it take her to die? A day? Two days?

It was no good. I had to do something about it. I ran out to my car, grabbed the bottle of nembutal and my big 50 c.c. syringe and hurried back into the stable. I vaulted over the rotting timbers of the door, drew out 40 c.c.'s from the bottle and plunged the whole dose into the sheep's peritoneal cavity. Then I leapt back, galloped the length of the stable and when Mr Kitson returned I was standing innocently where he had left me.

I towelled myself, put on my jacket and gathered up my bottle of antiseptic and the tube of cream which had served me so well.

Mr Kitson preceded me along the stable and on the way out he glanced over the door in the corner.

'By gaw, she's goin' fast,' he grunted.

I looked over his shoulder into the gloom. The panting had stopped and was replaced by slow, even respirations. The eyes were closed. The sheep was anaesthetised. She would die in peace.

'Yes,' I said. 'She's definitely sinking. I don't think it will be very long now.' I couldn't resist a parting shaft. 'You've lost this ewe and that lamb back there. I think I could have saved both of them for you if you'd given me a chance.'

Maybe my words got through to Mr Kitson, because I was surprised to be called back to the farm a few days later to a ewe which had obviously suffered very little interference.

The animal was in a field close to the house and she was clearly bursting with lambs; so round and fat she could hardly waddle. But she looked bright and healthy.

'There's a bloody mix-up in there,' Mr Kitson said morosely. 'Ah could feel two heads and God only knows how many feet. Didn't know where the 'ell I was.'

'But you didn't try very hard?'

'Nay, never tried at all.'

Well, we were making progress. As the farmer gripped the sheep round the neck I knelt behind her and dipped my hands in the bucket. For once it was a warm morning. Looking back, my memories of lambing times have been of bitter winds searing the grass of the hill pastures, of chapped hands, chafed arms, gloves, scarves and cold-nipped ears. For years after I left Glasgow I kept waiting for the balmy early springs of western Scotland. After thirty years I am still waiting and it has begun to dawn on me that it doesn't happen that way in Yorkshire.

But this morning was one of the exceptions. The sun blazed from a sky of soft blue, there was no wind but a gentle movement of the air rolled the fragrance of the moorland flowers and warm grass over and around me as I knelt there.

And I had my favourite job in front of me. I almost chuckled as I fished around inside the ewe. There was all the room in the world, everything was moist and fresh and unspoiled, and it was child's play to fit the various jigsaws together. In about thirty seconds I had a lamb wriggling on the grass, in a few moments more a second, then a third and finally to my delight I reached away forward and found another little cloven foot and whisked it out into the world.

'Quadruplets!' I cried happily, but the farmer didn't share my enthusiasm.

'Nowt but a bloody nuisance,' he muttered. 'She'd be far better wi' just two.' He paused and gave me a sour look. 'Any road, ah reckon there wasn't no need to call ye. I could've done that job meself.'

I looked at him sadly from my squatting position. Sometimes in our job you feel you just can't win. If you take too long you're no good, if you're too quick the visit wasn't necessary. I have never quite subscribed to the views of a cynical old colleague who once adjured me: 'Never make a lambing look easy. Hold the buggers in for a few minutes if necessary.' But at times I felt he had a point.

Anyway, I had my own satisfaction in watching the four lambs. So often I had pitied these tiny creatures in their entry into an uncharitable world, sometimes even of snow and ice, but today it was a joy to see them trying to struggle to their feet under the friendly sun, their woolly coats already drying rapidly. Their mother, magically deflated, was moving among them in a bemused manner as though she couldn't quite believe what she saw. As she nosed and licked them her deep-throated chuckles were answered by the first treble quaverings of her family. I was listening, enchanted, to this conversation when Mr Kitson spoke up.

'There's t'ewe you lambed t'other day.'

I looked up and there indeed she was, trotting proudly past, her lamb close at her flank.

'Ah yes, she looks fine,' I said. That was good to see but my attention was caught by something else. I pointed across the grass.

'That ewe away over there . . .' As a rule all sheep look alike to me but there was something about this one I recognised . . . a loss of wool from her back, a bare strip of skin stretched over the jutting ridge of her spinal column . . . surely I couldn't be mistaken.

The farmer followed my pointing finger. 'Aye, that's t'awd lass that was laid in the stable last time you were here.' He turned an expressionless gaze on me. 'The one you told me to get Mallock to fetch.'

'But . . . but . . . she was dying!' I blurted out.

The corner of Mr Kitson's mouth twitched upwards in what must have been the nearest possible approach to a smile. 'Well, that's what you tellt me, young feller.' He hunched his shoulders. 'Said she 'adn't long to go, didn't you?'

I had no words to offer. I just gaped at him. I must have been the picture of bewilderment and it seemed the farmer was puzzled too because he went on.

'But I'll tell tha summat. Ah've been among sheep all me life but ah've never seen owt like it. That ewe just went to sleep.'

'Is that so?'

'Aye, went to sleep, ah tell you and she stayed sleepin' for two days!'

'She slept for two days?'

'She did, ah'm not jokin', nor jestin'. Ah kept goin' into t'stable but she never altered. Lay there peaceful as you like all

143

t'first day, then all t'second, then when I went in on t'third morning she was standin' there lookin' at me and ready for some grub.'

'Amazing!' I got to my feet. 'I must have a look at her.'

I really wanted to see what had become of that mass of inflammation and tumefaction under her tail and I approached her carefully, jockeying her bit by bit into the bottom corner of the field. There we faced each other for a few tense moments as I tried a few feints and she responded with nimble side-steps; then as I made my final swoop to catch her fleece she eluded me effortlessly and shot past me with a thundering of hooves. I gave chase for twenty yards but it was too hot and wellingtons aren't the ideal gear for running. In any case I have long held the notion that if a vet can't catch his patient there's nothing much to worry about.

And as I walked back up the field a message was tapping in my brain. I had discovered something, discovered something by accident. That ewe's life had been saved not by medicinal therapy but simply by stopping her pain and allowing nature to do its own job of healing. It was a lesson I have never forgotten; that animals confronted with severe continuous pain and the terror and shock that goes with it will often retreat even into death, and if you can remove that pain amazing things can happen. It is difficult to explain rationally but I know that it is so.

By the time I had got back to Mr Kitson the sun was scorching the back of my neck and I could feel a trickle of sweat under my shirt. The big man was still watching the ewe which had finished its gallop and was cropping the grass contentedly.

'Ah can't get over it,' he murmured, scratching the thin bristle on his jaw. 'Two whole days and never a move.' He turned to me and his eyes widened.

'Ah'll tell tha, young man, you'd just think she'd been drugged!'

21

I found it difficult to get Mr Kitson's ewe out of my mind but I had to make the effort because while all the sheep work was going on the rest of the practice problems rolled along unabated. One of these concerned the Flaxton's Poodle, Penny.

Penny's first visit to the surgery was made notable by the attractiveness of her mistress. When I stuck my head round the waiting-room door and said, 'Next please,' Mrs Flaxton's little round face with its shining tight cap of blue-black hair seemed to illuminate the place like a beacon. It is possible that the effect was heightened by the fact that she was sitting between fifteen stone Mrs Barmby, who had brought her canary to have its claws clipped, and old Mr Spence who was nearly ninety and had called round for some flea powder for his cat, but there was no doubt she was good to look at.

And it wasn't just that she was pretty; there was a round-eyed, innocent appeal about her and she smiled all the time. Penny, sitting on her knee, seemed to be smiling from under the mound of brown curls on her forehead.

In the consulting room I lifted the little dog on to the table. 'Well now, what's the trouble?'

'She has a touch of sickness and diarrhoea,' Mrs Flaxton replied. 'It started yesterday.'

'I see.' I turned and lifted the thermometer from the trolley. 'Has she had a change of food?'

'No, nothing like that.'

'Is she inclined to eat rubbish when she's out?'

Mrs Flaxton shook her head. 'No, not as a rule. But I suppose even the nicest dog will have a nibble at a dead bird or something horrid like that now and then.' She laughed and Penny laughed back at her.

'Well, she has a slightly raised temperature but she seems bright enough.' I put my hand round the dog's middle. 'Let's have a feel at your tummy, Penny.'

The little animal winced as I gently palpated the abdomen, and there was a tenderness throughout the stomach and intestines.

'She has gastroenteritis,' I said. 'But it seems fairly mild and I think it should clear up quite soon. I'll give you some medicine for her and you'd better keep her on a light diet for a few days.'

'Yes, I'll do that. Thank you very much.' Mrs Flaxton's smile deepened as she patted her dog's head. She was about twenty-three and she and her young husband had only recently come to Darrowby. He was a representative of one of the big agricultural firms which supplied meal and cattle cake to the farms and I saw him occasionally on my rounds. Like his wife, and indeed his dog, he gave off an ambience of eager friendliness.

I sent Mrs Flaxton off with a bottle of bismuth, kaolin and chlorodyne mixture which was one of our cherished treatments. The little dog trotted down the surgery steps, tail wagging, and I really didn't expect any more trouble.

Three days later, however, Penny was in the surgery again. She was still vomiting and the diarrhoea had not taken up in the least.

I got the dog on the table again and carried out a further examination but there was nothing significant to see. She had now had five days of this weakening condition but though she had lost a bit of her perkiness she still looked remarkably bright. The Toy Poodle is small but tough and very game and this one wasn't going to let anything get her down easily.

But I still didn't like it. She couldn't go on like this. I decided to alter the treatment to a mixture of carbon and astringents which had served me well in the past.

'This stuff looks a bit messy,' I said, as I gave Mrs Flaxton a powder box full of the black granules. 'But I have had good results with it. She's still eating, isn't she, so I should mix it in her food.'

'Oh thank you.' She gave me one of her marvellous smiles as she put the box in her bag and I walked along the passage with her to the door. She had left her pram at the foot of the steps and I knew before I looked under the hood what kind of baby

I would find. Sure enough the chubby face on the pillow gazed at me with round friendly eyes and then split into a delightful grin.

They were the kind of people I liked to see but as they moved off down the street I hoped for Penny's sake that I wouldn't be seeing them for a long time. However, it was not to be. A couple of days later they were back and this time the Poodle was showing signs of strain. As I examined her she stood motionless and dead-eyed with only the occasional twitch of her tail as I stroked her head and spoke to her.

'I'm afraid she's just the same, Mr Herriot,' her mistress said. 'She's not eating much now and whatever she does goes straight through her. And she has a terrific thirst – always at her water bowl and then she brings it back.'

I nodded. 'I know. This inflammation inside her gives her a raging desire for water and of course the more she drinks the more she vomits. And this is terribly weakening.'

Again I changed the treatment. In fact over the next few days I ran through just about the entire range of available drugs. I look back with a wry smile at the things I gave that little dog, powdered epicacuanha and opium, sodium salicylate and tincture of camphor, even way-out exotics like decoction of haematoxylin and infusion of caryophyllum which thank heavens have been long forgotten. I might have done a bit of good if I had had access to a gut-active antibiotic like neomycin but as it was I got nowhere.

I was visiting Penny daily as she was unfit to bring to the surgery. I had her on a diet of arrowroot and boiled milk but that, like my medical treatment, achieved nothing. And all the time the little dog was slipping away.

The climax came about three o'clock one morning. As I lifted the bedside phone Mr Flaxton's voice, with a tremor in it, came over the line.

'I'm terribly sorry to get you out of your bed at this hour, Mr Herriot, but I wish you'd come round to see Penny.'

'Why, is she worse?'

'Yes, and she's . . . well . . . she's suffering now, I'm afraid.

147

You saw her this afternoon, didn't you? Well since then she's been drinking and vomiting and this diarrhoea running away from her all the time till she's about at the far end. She's just lying in her basket crying. I'm sure she's in great pain.'

'Right, I'll be there in a few minutes.'

'Oh thank you.' He paused for a moment. 'And Mr Herriot ... you'll come prepared to put her down, won't you?'

My spirits, never very high at that time in the morning, plummeted to the depths. 'As bad as that, is it?'

'Well honestly we can't bear to see her. My wife is so upset ... I don't think she can stand any more.'

'I see.' I hung up the phone and threw the bedclothes back with a violence which brought Helen wide awake. Being disturbed in the small hours was one of the crosses a vet's wife has to bear, but normally I crept out as quietly as I could. This time, however, I stamped about the bedroom, dragging on my clothes and muttering to myself; and though she must have wondered what this latest crisis meant she wisely watched me in silence until I turned out the light and left.

I had not far to go. The Flaxtons lived in one of the new bungalows on the Brawton Road less than a mile away. The young couple, in their dressing gowns, led me into the kitchen and before I reached the dog basket in the corner I could hear Penny's whimperings. She was not lying comfortably curled up, but on her chest, head forward, obviously acutely distressed. I put my hands under her and lifted her and she was almost weightless. A Toy Poodle in its prime is fairly insubstantial but after her long illness Penny was like a bedraggled little piece of thistledown, her curly brown coat wet and soiled by vomit and diarrhoea.

Mrs Flaxton's smile for once was absent. I could see she was keeping back the tears as she spoke.

'It really would be the kindest thing . . .'

'Yes . . . yes . . .' I replaced the tiny animal in her basket and crouched over her, chin in hand. 'Yes, I suppose you're right.'

But still I didn't move but stayed, squatting there, staring down in disbelief at the evidence of my failure. This dog was only two years old – a lifetime of running and jumping and barking in front of her; all she was suffering from was gastroenteritis and now I was going to extinguish the final spark in her. It was a bitter thought that this would be just about the only positive thing I had done right from the start.

A weariness swept over me that was not just due to the fact that I had been snatched from sleep. I got to my feet with the slow stiff movements of an old man and was about to turn away when I noticed something about the little animal. She was on her chest again, head extended, mouth open, tongue lolling as she panted. There was something there I had seen before somewhere . . . that posture . . . and the exhaustion, pain and shock . . . it slid almost imperceptibly into my sleepy brain that she looked exactly like Mr Kitson's ewe in its dark corner. A different species, yes, but all the other things were there.

'Mrs Flaxton,' I said, 'I want to put Penny to sleep. Not the way you think, but to anaesthetise her. Maybe if she has a rest from this nonstop drinking and vomiting and straining it will give nature a chance.'

The young couple looked at me doubtfully for a few moments then it was the husband who spoke.

'Don't you think she has been through enough, Mr Herriot?'

'She has, yes she has.' I ran a hand through my rumpled uncombed hair. 'But this won't cause her any more distress. She won't know a thing about it.'

When they still hesitated I went on. 'I would very much like to try it – it's just an idea I've got.'

They looked at each other, then Mrs Flaxton nodded. 'All right, go ahead, but this will be the last, won't it?'

Out into the night air to my car for the same bottle of nembutal and a very small dose for the little creature. I went back to my bed with the same feeling I had had about the ewe; come what may there would be no more suffering.

Next morning Penny was still stretched peacefully on her side and when, about four o'clock in the afternoon, she showed signs of awakening I repeated the injection.

Like the ewe she slept for forty-eight hours and when she

finally did stagger to her feet she did not head immediately for her water bowl as she had done for so many days. Instead she made her feeble way outside and had a walk round the garden.

From then on, recovery, as they say in the case histories, was uneventful. Or as I would rather write it, she wonderfully and miraculously just got better and never ailed another thing throughout her long life.

Helen and I used to play tennis on the grass courts near the Darrowby cricket ground. So did the Flaxtons and they always brought Penny along with them. I used to look through the wire at her romping with other dogs and later with the Flaxtons' fast growing young son and I marvelled.

I do not wish to give the impression that I advocate wholesale anaesthesia for all animal ailments but I do know that sedation has a definite place. Nowadays we have a sophisticated range of sedatives and tranquillisers to choose from and when I come up against an acute case of gastroenteritis in dogs I use one of them as an adjunct to the normal treatment; because it puts a brake on the deadly exhausting cycle and blots out the pain and fear which go with it.

And over the years, whenever I saw Penny running around, barking, bright-eyed, full of the devil, I felt a renewed welling of thankfulness for the cure which I discovered in a dark corner of a stable by accident.

22

The name was on the garden gate – Lilac Cottage. I pulled out my list of visits and checked the entry again. 'Cook, Lilac Cottage, Marston Hall. Bitch overdue for whelping.' This was the place all right, standing in the grounds of the Hall, a nineteenth-century mansion house whose rounded turrets reared above the fringe of pine trees less than half a mile away.

The door was opened by a heavy featured dark woman of about sixty who regarded me unsmilingly.

'Good morning, Mrs Cook,' I said. 'I've come to see your bitch.'

She still didn't smile. 'Oh, very well. You'd better come in.'

She led me into the small living room and as a little Yorkshire Terrier jumped down from an armchair her manner changed.

'Come here, Cindy my darlin',' she cooed. 'This gentleman's come to make you better.' She bent down and stroked the little animal, her face radiant with affection.

I sat down in another armchair. 'Well what's the trouble, Mrs Cook?'

'Oh, I'm worried to death.' She clasped her hands anxiously. 'She should have had her pups yesterday and there's nothing happenin'. Ah couldn't sleep all night – I'd die if anything happened to this dog.'

I looked at the terrier, tail wagging, gazing up, bright-eyed under her mistress's caress. 'She doesn't seem distressed at all. Has she shown any signs of labour?'

'What d'you mean?'

'Well, has she been panting or uneasy in any way? Is there any discharge?'

'No, nothing like that.'

I beckoned to Cindy and spoke to her and she came timidly across the lino till I was able to lift her on to my lap. I palpated the distended abdomen; there were a lot of pups in there but everything appeared normal. I took her temperature – normal again.

'Bring me some warm water and soap, Mrs Cook, will you please?' I said. The terrier was so small that I had to use my little finger, soaped and disinfected, to examine her, and as I felt carefully forward the walls of the vagina were dry and clinging and the cervix, when I reached it, tightly closed.

I washed and dried my hands. 'This little bitch isn't anywhere near whelping, Mrs Cook. Are you sure you haven't got your dates wrong?'

'No, I 'aven't, it was sixty-three days yesterday.' She paused in thought for a moment. 'Now ah'd better tell you this, young man. Cindy's had pups before and she did self and same thing – wouldn't get on with t'job. That was two years ago when I was livin' over in Listondale. I got Mr Broomfield the vet to her and he just gave her an injection. It was wonderful – she had the pups half an hour after it.'

I smiled. 'Yes, that would be pituitrin. She must have been actually whelping when Mr Broomfield saw her.'

'Well whatever it was, young man, I wish you'd give her some now. Ah can't stand all this suspense.'

'I'm sorry.' I lifted Cindy from my lap and stood up. 'I can't do that. It would be very harmful at this stage.'

She stared at me and it struck me that that dark face could look very forbidding. 'So you're not goin' to do anything at all?'

'Well . . .' There are times when it is a soothing procedure to give a client something to do even if it is unnecessary. 'Yes, I've got some tablets in the car. They'll help to keep the little dog fit until she whelps.'

'But I'd far rather have that injection. It was just a little prick. Didn't take Mr Broomfield more than a second to do.'

'I assure you, Mrs Cook, it can't be done at the moment. I'll get the tablets from the car.'

Her mouth tightened. I could see she was grievously disappointed in me. 'Oh well if you won't you won't, so you'd better get them things.' She paused: 'And me name isn't Cook!'

'It isn't?'

'No it isn't, young man.' She didn't seem disposed to offer further information so I left in some bewilderment.

Out in the road, a few yards from my car, a farm man was trying to start a tractor. I called over to him.

'Hey, the lady in there says her name isn't Cook.'

'She's right an' all. She's the cook over at the Hall. You've gotten a bit mixed up.' He laughed heartily.

It all became suddenly clear; the entry in the day book, everything. 'What's her right name, then?'

'Booby,' he shouted just as the tractor roared into life.

Funny name, I thought, as I produced my harmless vitamin tablets from the boot and returned to the cottage. Once inside I did my best to put things right with plenty of 'Yes, Mrs Booby' and 'No, Mrs Booby' but the lady didn't thaw. I told her not to worry and that I was sure nothing would happen for several days but I could tell I wasn't impressing her.

I waved cheerfully as I went down the path.

'Goodbye, Mrs Booby,' I cried. 'Don't hesitate to ring me if you're in doubt about anything.'

She didn't appear to have heard.

'Oh I wish you'd do as I say,' she wailed. 'It was just a little prick.'

The good lady certainly didn't hesitate to ring. She was at me again the next day and I had to rush out to her cottage. Her message was the same as before; she wanted the wonderful injection which would make those pups pop out and she wanted it right away. Mr Broomfield hadn't messed about and wasted time like I had. And on the third and fourth and fifth mornings she had me out at Marston examining the little bitch and reciting the same explanations. Things came to a head on the sixth day.

In the room at Lilac Cottage the dark eyes held a desperate light as they stared into mine. 'I'm about at the end of my tether, young man. I tell you I'll die if anything happens to this dog. I'll die. Don't you understand?'

'Of course I know how you feel about her, Mrs Booby. Believe me, I fully understand.'

'Then why don't you do something?' she snapped.

I dug my nails into my palms. 'Look, I've told you. A pituitrin injection works by contracting the muscular walls of the uterus, so it can only be given when labour has started and the cervix is open. If I find it is indicated I will do it, but if I give this injection now it could cause rupture of the uterus. It could cause death.' I stopped because I fancied little bubbles were beginning to collect at the corners of my mouth.

But I don't think she had listened to a word. She sunk her head in her hands. 'All this time, I can't stand it.'

I was wondering if I could stand more of it myself. Bulging Yorkshire Terriers had begun to prance through my dreams at night and I greeted each new day with a silent prayer that the pups had arrived. I held out my hand to Cindy and she crept reluctantly towards me. She was heartily sick of this strange man who came every day and squeezed her and stuck fingers into her and she submitted again with trembling limbs and frightened eyes to the indignity.

'Mrs Booby,' I said, 'are you absolutely sure that dog didn't have access to Cindy after the service date you gave me?'

She sniffed. 'You keep askin' me that and ah've been thinking about it. Maybe he did come a week after, now I think on.'

'Well, that's it, then!' I spread my hands. 'She's held to the second mating, so she should be due tomorrow.'

'Ah would still far rather you would get it over with today like Mr Broomfield did . . . it was just a little prick.'

'But Mrs Booby . . .!'

'And let me tell you another thing, me name's not Booby!'

I clutched at the back of the chair. 'It's not?'

'Naw!'

'Well . . . what is it, then?'

'It's Dooley . . . Dooley!' She looked very cross.

'Right . . . right . . .' I stumbled down the garden path and drove away. It was not a happy departure.

Next morning I could hardly believe it when there was no call from Marston. Maybe all was well at last. But I turned cold when an urgent call to go to Lilac Cottage was passed on to one of the farms on my round. I was right at the far end of the practice area and was in the middle of a tough calving and it was well over three hours before I got out at the now familiar garden gate. The cottage door was open and as I ventured up the path a little brown missile hurtled out at me. It was Cindy, but a transformed Cindy, a snarling, barking little bundle of ferocity; and though I recoiled she fastened her teeth in my trouser cuff and hung on grimly.

I was hopping around on one leg trying to shake off the growling little creature when a peal of almost girlish laughter made me look round.

Mrs Dooley, vastly amused, was watching me from the doorway. 'My word, she's different since she had them pups. Just shows what a good little mother she is, guarding them like that.' She gazed fondly at the tiny animal dangling from my ankle.

'Had the pups . . . ?'

'Aye, when they said you'd be a long time I rang Mr Farnon. He came right away and d'you know he gave Cindy that injection I've wanted all along. And I tell you 'e wasn't right out of t'garden gate before the pups started. She's had seven – beauties they are.'

'Ah well that's fine, Mrs Dooley . . . splendid.' Siegfried had obviously felt a pup in the passage. I finally managed to rid myself of Cindy and when her mistress lifted her up I went into the kitchen to inspect the family.

They certainly were grand pups and I lifted the squawking little morsels one by one from their basket while their mother snarled from Mrs Dooley's arms like a starving wolfhound.

'They're lovely, Mrs Dooley,' I murmured.

She looked at me pityingly. 'I told you what to do, didn't I, but you wouldn't 'ave it. It only needed a little prick. Ooo, that Mr Farnon's a lovely man – just like Mr Broomfield.'

This was a bit much. 'But you must realise, Mrs Dooley, he just happened to arrive at the right time. If I had come . . .'

'Now, now, young man, be fair. Ah'm not blamin' you, but some people have had more experience. We all 'ave to learn.' She sighed reminiscently. 'It was just a little prick – Mr Farnon'll have to show you how to do it. I tell you he wasn't right out of t'garden gate . . .'

Enough is enough. I drew myself up to my full height. 'Mrs Dooley, madam,' I said frigidly, 'let me repeat once and for all . . .'

'Oh, hoity toity, hoity toity, don't get on your high horse wi' me!' she exclaimed. 'We've managed very nicely without you, so don't complain.' Her expression became very severe. 'And one more thing – me name's not Mrs Dooley.'

My brain reeled for a moment. The world seemed to be crumbling about me. 'What did you say?'

'I said me name's not Mrs Dooley.'

'It isn't?'

'Naw!' She lifted her left hand and as I gazed at it dully I realised it must have been all the mental stress which had prevented me from noticing the total absence of rings.

'Naw!' she said. 'It's Miss!'

23

I had never been married before so there was nothing in my past experience to go by but it was beginning to dawn on me that I was very nicely fixed.

I am talking, of course, of material things. It would have been enough for me or anybody else to be paired with a beautiful girl whom I loved and who loved me. I hadn't reckoned on the other aspects.

This business of studying my comfort, for instance. I thought such things had gone out of fashion, but not so with Helen. It was brought home to me again as I walked in to breakfast this morning. We had at last acquired a table – I had bought it at a farm sale and brought it home in triumph tied to the roof of my car – and now Helen had vacated the chair on which she used to sit at the bench and had taken over the high stool. She was perched away up there now, transporting her food from far below, while I was expected to sit comfortably in the chair. I don't think I am a selfish swine by nature but there was nothing I could do about it.

And there were other little things. The neat pile of clothing laid out for me each morning; the clean, folded shirt and hand-kerchief and socks so different from the jumble of my bachelor days. And when I was late for meals, which was often, she served me with my food but instead of going off and doing something else she would down tools and sit watching me while I ate. It made me feel like a sultan.

It was this last trait which gave me a clue to her behaviour. I suddenly remembered that I had seen her sitting by Mr Alderson while he had a late meal; sitting in the same pose, one arm on the table, quietly watching him. And I realised I was reaping the benefit of her lifetime attitude to her father. Mild little man though he was she had catered gladly to his every wish in the happy acceptance that the man of the house was number one; and the whole pattern was rubbing off on me now.

In fact it set me thinking about the big question of how girls might be expected to behave after marriage. One old farmer giving me advice about choosing a wife once said; 'Have a bloody good look at the mother first, lad', and I am sure he had a point. But if I may throw in my own little word of counsel it would be to have a passing glance at how she acts towards her father.

Watching her now as she got down and started to serve my breakfast the warm knowledge flowed through me as it did so often that my wife was the sort who just liked looking after a man and that I was so very lucky.

And I was certainly blooming under the treatment. A bit too much, in fact, and I was aware I shouldn't be attacking this plateful of porridge and cream; especially with all that material sizzling in the frying pan. Helen had brought with her to Skel-dale House a delicious dowry in the shape of half a pig and there hung from the beams of the topmost attic a side of bacon and a majestic ham; a constant temptation. Some samples were in the pan now and though I had never been one for large breakfasts I did not demur when she threw in a couple of big brown eggs to keep them company. And I put up only feeble resistance when she added some particularly tasty smoked sausage which she used to buy in a shop in the market place.

When I had got through it all I rose rather deliberately from the table and as I put on my coat I noticed it wasn't so easy to button as it used to be.

'Here are your sandwiches, Jim,' Helen said, putting a parcel in my hand. I was spending a day in the Scarburn district, tuberculin testing for Ewan Ross, and my wife was always concerned lest I grow faint from lack of nourishment on the long journey.

I kissed her, made a somewhat ponderous descent of the long flights of stairs and went out the side door. Half way up the garden I stopped as always and looked up at the window under the tiles. An arm appeared and brandished a dishcloth vigorously. I waved back and continued my walk to the yard. I found I was puffing a little as I got the car out and I laid my parcel almost guiltily on the back seat. I knew what it would contain; not just sandwiches but meat and onion pie, buttered scones, ginger cake to lead me into further indiscretions.

There is no doubt that in those early days I would have grown exceedingly gross under Helen's treatment. But my job saved me; the endless walking between the stone barns scattered along the hillsides, the climbing in and out of calf pens, pushing cows around, and regular outbursts of hard physical effort in calving and foaling. So I escaped with only a slight tightening of my collar and the occasional farmer's remark, 'By gaw, you've been on a good pasture, young man!'

Driving away, I marvelled at the way she indulged my little whims, too. I have always had a pathological loathing of fat, so Helen carefully trimmed every morsel from my meat. This feeling about fat, which almost amounted to terror, had been intensified since coming to Yorkshire, because back in the thirties the farmers seemed to live on the stuff. One old man, noticing my pop-eyed expression as I viewed him relishing his lunch of roast fat bacon, told me he had never touched lean meat in his life.

'Ah like to feel t'grease runnin' down ma chin!' he chuckled. He pronounced it 'grayus' which made it sound even worse. But he was a ruddy-faced octogenarian, so it hadn't done him any harm; and this held good for hundreds of others just like him. I used to think that the day in day out hard labour of farming burned it up in their systems but if I had to eat the stuff it would kill me very rapidly.

The latter was, of course, a fanciful notion as was proved to me one day.

It was when I was torn from my bed one morning at 6 a.m. to attend a calving heifer at old Mr Horner's small farm and when I got there I found there was no malpresentation of the calf but that it was simply too big. I don't like a lot of pulling but the heifer, lying on her bed of straw, was obviously in need of assistance. Every few seconds she strained to the utmost and a pair of feet came into view momentarily then disappeared as she relaxed.

'Is she getting those feet out any further?' I asked.

'Nay, there's been no change for over an hour,' the old man replied.

'And when did the water bag burst?'

'Two hours since.'

There was no doubt the calf was well and truly stuck and getting drier all the time, and if the labouring mother had been able to speak I think she would have said: 'For Pete's sake get this thing away from me!'

I could have done with a big strong man to help me but Mr Horner, apart from his advanced age, was a rather shaky lightweight. And since the farm was perched on a lonely eminence miles from the nearest village there was no chance of calling in a neighbour. I would have to do the job myself.

It took me nearly an hour. With a thin rope behind the calf's ears and through his mouth to stop the neck from telescoping I eased the little creature inch by inch into the world. Not so much pulling but rather leaning back and helping the heifer as she strained. She was a rather undersized little animal and she lay patiently on her side, accepting the situation with the resignation of her kind. She could never have calved without help and all the time I had the warm conviction that I was doing what she wanted and needed. I felt I should be as patient as she was so I didn't hurry but let things come in their normal sequence; the little nose with the nostrils twitching reassuringly, then the eyes wearing a preoccupied light during the tight squeeze, then the ears and with a final rush the rest of the calf.

The young mother was obviously none the worse because she rolled on to her chest almost immediately and began to sniff with the utmost interest at the new arrival. She was in better shape than myself because I discovered with some surprise that I was sweating and breathless and my arms and shoulders were aching.

The farmer, highly pleased, rubbed my back briskly with the towel as I bent over the bucket, then he helped me on with my shirt.

'Well that's champion, lad. You'll come in and have a cup of tea now, won't you?'

In the kitchen Mrs Horner placed a steaming mug on the table and smiled across at me.

'Will you sit down along o' my husband and have a bit o' breakfast?' she asked.

There is nothing like an early calving to whet the appetite and I nodded readily. 'That's very kind of you, I'd love to.'

It is always a good feeling after a successful delivery and I sighed contentedly as I sank into a chair and watched the old lady set out bread, butter and jam in front of me. I sipped my tea and as I exchanged a word with the farmer I didn't see what she was doing next. Then my toes curled into a tight ball as I found two huge slices of pure white fat lying on my plate.

Shrinking back in my seat I saw Mrs Horner sawing at a great hunk of cold boiled bacon. But it wasn't ordinary bacon, it was one hundred per cent fat without a strip of lean anywhere. Even in my shocked state I could see it was a work of art; cooked to a turn, beautifully encrusted with golden crumbs and resting on a spotless serving dish . . . but fat.

She dropped two similar slices on her husband's plate and looked at me expectantly.

My position was desperate. I could not possibly offend this

sweet old person but on the other hand I knew beyond all doubt that there was no way I could eat what lay in front of me. Maybe I could have managed a tiny piece if it had been hot and fried crisp, but cold, boiled and clammy . . . never. And there was an enormous quantity; two slices about six inches by four and at least half an inch thick with the golden border of crumbs down one side. The thing was impossible.

Mrs Horner sat down opposite me. She was wearing a flowered mob cap over her white hair and for a moment she reached out, bent her head to one side and turned the dish with the slab of bacon a little to the left to show it off better. Then she turned to me and smiled. It was a kind, proud smile.

There have been times in my life when, confronted by black and hopeless circumstances, I have discovered in myself un-dreamed-of resources of courage and resolution. I took a deep breath, seized knife and fork and made a bold incision in one of the slices, but as I began to transport the greasy white segment to my mouth I began to shudder and my hand stayed frozen in space. It was at that moment I spotted the jar of piccalilli.

Feverishly I scooped a mound of it on to my plate. It seemed to contain just about everything; onions, apples, cucumber and other assorted vegetables jostling each other in a powerful mustard-vinegar sauce. It was the work of a moment to smother my loaded fork with the mass, then I popped it into my mouth, gave a couple of quick chews and swallowed. It was a start and I hadn't tasted a thing except the piccalilli.

'Nice bit of bacon,' Mr Horner murmured.

'Delicious!' I replied, munching desperately at the second forkful. 'Absolutely delicious!'

'And you like ma piccalilli too!' The old lady beamed at me. 'Ah can tell by the way you're slappin' it on!' She gave a peal of delighted laughter.

'Yes, indeed.' I looked at her with streaming eyes. 'Some of the best I've ever tasted.'

Looking back, I realise it was one of the bravest things I have ever done. I stuck to my task unwaveringly, dipping again and again into the jar, keeping my mind a blank, refusing grimly to think of the horrible thing that was happening to me. There was only one bad moment, when the piccalilli, which packed a tremendous punch and was never meant to be consumed in large mouthfuls, completely took my breath away and I went into a long coughing spasm. But at last I came to the end. A final heroic crunch and swallow, a long gulp at my tea and the plate was empty. The thing was accomplished.

And there was no doubt it had been worth it. I had been a tremendous success with the old folks. Mr Horner slapped my shoulder.

'By gaw, it's good to see a young feller enjoyin' his food! When I were a lad I used to put it away sharpish, like that, but ah can't do it now.' Chuckling to himself, he continued with his breakfast.

His wife showed me the door. 'Aye, it was a real compliment to me.' She looked at the table and giggled. 'You've nearly finished the jar!'

'Yes, I'm sorry, Mrs Horner,' I said, smiling through my tears and trying to ignore the churning in my stomach. 'But I just couldn't resist it.'

Contrary to my expectations I didn't drop down dead soon afterwards but for a week I was oppressed by a feeling of nausea which I am prepared to believe was purely psychosomatic.

At any rate, since that little episode I have never knowingly eaten fat again. My hatred was transformed into something like an obsession from then on.

And I haven't been all that crazy about piccalilli either.

24

I wondered how long this feeling of novelty at being a married man would last. Maybe it went on for years and years. At any rate I did feel an entirely different person from the old Herriot as I paced with my wife among the stalls at the garden fête.

It was an annual affair in aid of the Society for the Prevention of Cruelty to Children and it was held on the big lawn behind the Darrowby vicarage with the weathered brick of the old house showing mellow red beyond the trees. The hot June sunshine bathed the typically English scene; the women in their flowered dresses, the men perspiring in their best suits, laughing children running from the tombola to the coconut shy or the ice-cream kiosk. In a little tent at one end, Mrs Newbould, the butcher's wife, thinly disguised as Madame Claire the fortune teller, was doing a brisk trade. It all seemed a long way from Glasgow.

And the solid citizen feeling was heightened by the pressure of Helen's hand on my arm and the friendly nods of the passers-by. One of these was the curate, Mr Blenkinsopp. He came up to us, exuding, as always, a charm that was completely unworldly.

'Ah, James,' he murmured. 'And Helen!' He beamed on us with the benevolence he felt for the entire human race. 'How nice to see you here!'

He walked along with us as the scent from the flower beds and the trodden grass rose in the warm air.

'You know, James, I was just thinking about you the other day. I was in Rainby – you know I take the service there every second week – and they were telling me they were having great difficulty in finding young men for the cricket team. I wondered if you would care to turn out for them.'

'Me? Play cricket?'

'Yes, of course.'

I laughed. 'I'm afraid I'm no cricketer. I'm interested in the game and I like to watch it, but where I come from they don't play it very much.'

'Oh, but surely you must have played at some time or other.'

'A bit at school, but they go more for tennis in Scotland. And anyway it was a long time ago.'

'Oh well, there you are.' Mr Blenkinsopp spread his hands. 'It will come back to you easily.'

'I don't know about that,' I said. 'But another thing, I don't live in Rainby, doesn't that matter?'

'Not really,' the curate replied. 'It is such a problem finding eleven players in these tiny villages that they often call on outsiders. Nobody minds.'

I stopped my stroll over the grass and turned to Helen. She was giving me an encouraging smile and I began to think, well . . . why not? It looked as though I had settled in Yorkshire. I had married a Yorkshire girl. I might as well start doing the Yorkshire things, like playing cricket – there wasn't anything more Yorkshire than that.

'All right then, Mr Blenkinsopp,' I said. 'You're not getting any bargain but I don't mind having a go.'

'Splendid! The next match is on Tuesday evening – against Hedwick. I am playing so I'll pick you up at six o'clock.' His face radiated happiness as though I had done him the greatest favour.

'Well, thanks,' I replied. 'I'll have to fix it with my partner to be off that night, but I'm sure it will be O.K.'

The weather was still fine on Tuesday and, going round my visits, I found it difficult to assimilate the fact that for the first time in my life I was going to perform in a real genuine cricket match.

It was funny the way I felt about cricket. All my experience of the game was based on the long-range impressions I had gained during my Glasgow boyhood. Gleaned from newspapers, from boys' magazines, from occasional glimpses of Hobbs and Sutcliffe and Woolley on the cinema newsreels, they had built up a strangely glamorous picture in my mind. The whole thing, it seemed to me, was so deeply and completely English; the gentle clunk of bat on ball, the white-clad figures on the wide sweep of smooth turf; there was a softness, a graciousness about cricket which you found nowhere else; nobody ever got excited or upset at this leisurely pursuit. There was no doubt at all that I looked on cricket with a romanticism and nostalgia which would have been incomprehensible to people who had played the game all their lives.

Promptly at six Mr Blenkinsopp tooted the horn of his little car outside the surgery. Helen had advised me to dress ready for action and she had clearly been right because the curate, too, was resplendent in white flannels and blazer. The three young farmers crammed in the back were, however, wearing open-necked shirts with their ordinary clothes.

'Hello, James!' said Mr Blenkinsopp.

'Now then, Jim,' said two of the young men in the back. But 'Good afternoon, Mr Herriot,' said the one in the middle.

He was Tom Willis, the captain of the Rainby team and in my opinion, one of nature's gentlemen. He was about my own age and he and his father ran the kind of impoverished small-holding which just about kept them alive. But there was a sen-sitivity and refinement about him and a courtesy which never varied. I never cared how people addressed me and a lot of the farmers used my first name, but to Tom and his father I was always Mr Herriot. They considered it was the correct way to address the vet and that was that.

Tom leaned from the back seat now, his lean face set in its usual serious expression.

'It's good of you to give up your time, Mr Herriot. I know you're a busy man but we're allus short o' players at Rainby.'

'I'm looking forward to it, Tom, but I'm no cricketer, I'll tell you now.'

He gazed at me with gentle disbelief and I had an uncomfort-able feeling that everybody had the impression that because I had been to college I was bound to have a blue.

Hedwick was at the top end of Allerdale, a smaller offshoot of the main Dale, and as we drove up the deep ever-narrowing cleft in the moorland I wound down the window. It was the sort of country I saw every day but I wasn't used to being a passenger and there was no doubt you could see more this way. From the overlapping fringe of heather far above, the walls ran in spidery lines down the bare green flanks to the softness of the valley floor where grey farmhouses crouched; and the heavy scent of the new cut hay lying in golden swathes in the meadows drifted into the car. There were trees, too, down here, not the stunted dwarfs of the high country above us, but giants in the exultant foliage of high summer.

We stopped at Hedwick because we could go no further. This was the head of the Dale, a cluster of cottages, a farm and a pub. Where the road curved a few cars were drawn up by the side of a solid-looking wall on which leaned a long row of cloth-capped men, a few women and chattering groups of children.

'Ah,' said Mr Blenkinsopp. 'A good turn-out of spectators. Hedwick always support their team well. They must have come from all over the Dale.'

I looked around in surprise. 'Spectators?'

'Yes, of course. They've come to see the match.'

Again I gazed about me. 'But I can't see the pitch.'

'It's there,' Tom said. 'Just over t'wall.'

I leaned across the rough stones and stared in some bewilderment at a wildly undulating field almost knee deep in rough grass among which a cow, some sheep and a few hens wandered contentedly. 'Is this it?'

'Aye, that's it. If you stand on t'wall you can see the square.'

I did as he said and could just discern a five foot wide strip of bright green cut from the crowding herbage. The stumps stood expectantly at either end. A massive oak tree sprouted from somewhere around mid-on.

The strip stood on the only level part of the field, and that was a small part. Within twenty yards it swept up steeply to a thick wood which climbed over the lower slopes of the fell. On the other side it fell away to a sort of ravine where the rank grass ended only in a rocky stream. The wall bordering the near side ran up to a group of farm buildings.

There was no clubhouse but the visiting team were seated on a form on the grass while nearby, a little metal score board about four feet high stood near its pile of hooked number plates.

The rest of our team had arrived, too, and with a pang of alarm I noticed that there was not a single pair of white flannels among them. Only the curate and I were properly attired and the immediate and obvious snag was that he could play and I couldn't.

Tom and the home captain tossed a coin. Hedwick won and elected to bat. The umpires, two tousle-haired, sunburnt young fellows in grubby white coats strolled to the wicket, our team followed and the Hedwick batsmen appeared. Under their pads they wore navy blue serge trousers (a popular colour among both teams) and one of them sported a bright yellow sweater.

Tom Willis with the air of authority and responsibility which was natural to him began to dispose the field. No doubt convinced that I was a lynx-eyed catcher he stationed me quite close to the bat on the off side then after a grave consultation with Mr Blenkinsopp he gave him the ball and the game was on.

And Mr Blenkinsopp was a revelation. In his university sweater, gleaming flannels and brightly coloured cap he really looked good. And indeed it was soon very clear that he was good. He handed his cap to the umpire, retreated about twenty yards into the undergrowth, then turned and, ploughing his way back at ever increasing speed, delivered the ball with remarkable velocity bang on the wicket. The chap in yellow met it respectfully with a dead bat and did the same with the next but then he uncoiled himself and belted the third one high over the fielders on to the slope beneath the wood. As one of our men galloped after it the row of heads above the wall broke into a babel of noise.

They cheered every hit, not with the decorous ripple of applause I had always imagined, but with raucous yells. And they had plenty to shout about. The Hedwick lads, obviously accustomed to the peculiarities of their pitch wasted no time on classical strokes; they just gave a great hoick at the ball and when they connected it travelled immense distances. Occasionally they missed and Mr Blenkinsopp or one of our other bowlers shattered their stumps but the next man started cheerfully where they left off.

It was exhilarating stuff but I was unable to enjoy it. Everything I did, in fact my every movement proclaimed my ignorance to the knowledgeable people around me. I threw the ball in to the wrong end, I left the ball when I should have chased it and sped after it when I should have stayed in my place. I couldn't understand half the jargon which was being bandied around. No, there was not a shadow of a doubt about it; here in this cricket mad corner of a cricket mad county I was a foreigner.

Five wickets had gone down when a very fat lad came out to bat. His appearance of almost perfect rotundity was accentuated by the Fair Isle sweater stretched tightly over his bulging abdomen and judging by the barrage of witticisms which came from the heads along the wall it seemed he was a local character. He made a violent cross-batted swish at the first delivery, missed, and the ball sank with a thud into his midriff. Howls of laughter arose from players, spectators and umpires alike as he collapsed slowly at the crease and massaged himself ruefully. He slashed at the next one and it flew off the edge of his bat like a bullet, struck my shinbone a fearful crack and dropped into the grass. Resisting the impulse to scream and hop around in my agony I gritted my teeth, grabbed the ball and threw it in.

'Oh well stopped, Mr Herriot,' Tom Willis called from his position at mid-on. He clapped his hands a few times in encouragement.

Despite his girth the fat lad smote lustily and was finally caught in the outfield for fifteen.

The next batsman seemed to be taking a long time to reach the wicket. He was shuffling, bent-kneed, through the clover like a very old man, trailing his bat wearily behind him, and when he finally arrived at the crease I saw that he was indeed fairly advanced in years. He wore only one pad, strapped over baggy grey trousers which came almost up to his armpits and were suspended by braces. A cloth cap surmounted a face shrunken like a sour apple. From one corner of the downturned mouth a cigarette dangled.

He took guard and looked at the umpire.

'Middle and leg,' he grunted.

'Aye, that's about it, Len,' the umpire replied.

Len pursed his little mouth.

'About it . . . about it . . . ? Well is it or bloody isn't it ?' he enquired peevishly.

The young man in white grinned indulgently. 'Aye it is, Len, that's it.'

The old man removed his cigarette, flicked it on to the grass and took up his guard again. His appearance suggested that he might be out first ball or in fact that he had no right to be there at all, but as the delivery came down he stepped forward and with a scything sweep thumped the ball past the bowler and just a few inches above the rear end of the cow which had wandered into the line of fire. The animal looked round in some surprise as the ball whizzed along its backbone and the old man's crabbed features relaxed into the semblance of a smile.

'By gaw, vitnery,' he said, looking at me, 'ah damn near made a bit of work for tha there.' He eyed me impassively for a moment. 'Ah reckon tha's never took a cricket ball out of a cow's arse afore, eh ?'

Len returned to the job in hand and proved a difficult man to dislodge. But it was the batsman at the other end who was worrying Tom Willis. He had come in first wicket down, a ruddy faced lad of about nineteen wearing a blue shirt and he was still there piling on the runs.

At the end of the over, Tom came up to me. 'Fancy turning your arm over, Mr Herriot ?' he enquired gravely.

'Huh ?'

'Would you like a bowl ? A fresh man might just unsettle this feller.'

'Well . . . er . . .' I didn't know what to say. The idea of me bowling in a real match was unthinkable. Tom made up my mind by throwing me the ball.

Clasping it in a clammy hand I trotted up to the wicket while the lad in the blue shirt crouched intently over his bat. All the other bowlers had hurled their missiles down at top speed but as I ambled forward it burst on me that if I tried that I would be miles off my target. Accuracy, I decided, must be my watchword and I sent a gentle lob in the direction of the wicket. The batsman, obviously convinced that such a slow ball must be laden with hidden malice followed its course with deep suspicion and smothered it as soon as it arrived. He did the same with the second but that was enough for him to divine that I wasn't bowling off breaks, leg breaks or googlies but simply little dollies and he struck the third ball smartly into the ravine.

There was a universal cry of '*Maurice!*' from our team because Maurice Briggs, the Rainby blacksmith, was fielding down there and since he couldn't see the wicket he had to be warned. In due course the ball soared back from the depths, propelled no doubt by Maurice's strong right arm, and I recommenced my attack. The lad in blue thumped my remaining three deliveries effortlessly for six. The first flew straight over the wall and the row of cars into the adjoining field, the next landed in the farmyard and the third climbed in a tremendous arc away above the ravine and I heard it splash into the beck whence it was retrieved with a certain amount of profanity by the invisible Maurice.

An old farm man once said to me when describing a moment of embarrassment, 'Ah could've got down a mouse 'ole.' And as I returned to my place in the field I knew just what he meant. In fact the bowler at the other end got through his over almost without my noticing it and I was still shrunk in my cocoon of shame when I saw Tom Willis signalling to me.

I couldn't believe it. He was throwing me the ball again. It was a typically magnanimous gesture, a generous attempt to assure me that I had done well enough to have another go.

Again I shambled forward and the blue-shirted lad awaited me, almost licking his lips. He had never come across anyone like me before and it seemed too good to be true that I should be given another over; but there I was, and he climbed gratefully into each ball I sent down and laid into it in a kind of ecstasy with the full meat of the bat.

I would rather not go into details. Sufficient to say that I have a vivid memory of his red face and blue shirt and of the ball whistling back over my head after each delivery and of the almost berserk yells of the spectators. But he didn't hit every ball for six. In fact there were two moments of light relief in my torment; one when the ball smashed into the oak tree, ricocheted and almost decapitated old Len at the other end; the other when a ball snicked off the edge of the bat and ploughed through a very large cow pat, sending up a noisome spray along its course. It finished at the feet of Mr Blenkinsopp and the poor man was clearly in a dilemma. For the last hour he had been swooping on everything that came near him with the grace of the born cricketer.

But now he hovered over the unclean object, gingerly extending a hand then withdrawing it as his earthier colleagues in the team watched in wonder. The batsmen were galloping up and down, the crowd was roaring but the curate made no move. Finally he picked the thing up with the utmost daintiness in two fingers, regarded it distastefully for a few moments and carried it to the wicketkeeper who was ready with a handful of grass in his big gloves.

At the end of the over Tom came up to me. 'Thank ye, Mr Herriot, but I'm afraid I'll have to take you off now. This wicket's not suited to your type of bowling – not takin' spin at all.' He shook his head in his solemn way.

I nodded thankfully and Tom went on. 'Tell ye what, go down and relieve that man in the outfield. We could do wi' a safe pair of hands down there.'

25

I obeyed my skipper's orders and descended to the ravine and when Maurice had clambered up the small grassy cliff which separated me from the rest of the field I felt strangely alone. It was a dank, garlic-smelling region, perceptively colder than the land above and silent except for the gurgle of the beck behind me. There was a little hen house down here with several hens pecking around and some sheep who obviously felt it was safer than the higher ground.

I could see nothing of the pitch, only occasional glimpses of the heads of players so I had no idea of what was going on. In fact it was difficult to believe I was still taking part in a cricket match but for the spectators. From their position along the wall they had a grandstand view of everything and in fact were looking down at me from short range. They appeared to find me quite interesting, too, because a lot of them kept their eyes on me, puffing their pipes and making remarks which I couldn't hear but which caused considerable hilarity.

It was a pity about the spectators because it was rather peaceful in the ravine. It took a very big hit to get down there and I was more or less left to ruminate. Occasionally the warning cries would ring out from above and a ball would come bounding over the top. Once a skied drive landed with a thud in a patch of deep grass and with an enraged squawking a Rhode Island cockerel emerged at top speed and legged it irascibly to a safer haven.

Now and then I clawed my way up the bank and had a look at the progress of the game. Len had gone but the lad in blue was still there. After another dismissal I was surprised to see one of the umpires give his coat to the outgoing batsman, seize the bat and start laying about him. Both umpires were in fact members of the team.

It was after a long spell of inaction and when I was admiring the long splash of gold which the declining sun was throwing down the side of the fell when I heard the frantic yells. *'Jim ! James ! Mr Herriot !'* The whole team was giving tongue and, as I learned later, the lad in the blue shirt had made a catchable shot.

But I knew anyway. Nobody but he could have struck the blow which sent that little speck climbing higher and higher into the pale evening sky above me; and as it began with terrifying slowness to fall in my direction time came to a halt. I was aware of several of my team mates breasting the cliff and watching me breathlessly, of the long row of heads above the wall, and suddenly I was gripped by a cold resolve. I was going to catch this fellow out. He had humiliated me up there but it was my turn now.

The speck was coming down faster now as I stumbled about in the tangled vegetation trying to get into position. I nearly fell over a ewe with two big fat lambs sucking at her then I was right under the ball, hands cupped, waiting.

It fell, at the end, like a cannon ball, heavy and unyielding, on the end of my right thumb, bounded over my shoulder and thumped mournfully on the turf.

A storm of derision broke from the heads, peals of delighted laughter, volleys of candid comment.

'Get a basket!' advised one worthy.

'Fetch 'im a bucket!' suggested another.

As I scrabbled for the ball among the herbage I didn't know which was worse – the physical pain which was excruciating, or the mental anguish. After I had finally hurled the thing up the cliff I cradled the throbbing thumb in my other hand and rocked back and forth on my heels, moaning softly.

My team mates returned sadly to their tasks but Tom Willis, I noticed, lingered on, looking down at me.

'Hard luck, Mr Herriot. Very easy to lose t'ball against them trees.' He nodded encouragingly then was gone.

I was not troubled further in the innings. We never did get blue-shirt out and he had an unbeaten sixty-two at the close. The Hedwick score was a hundred and fifty-four, a very useful total in village cricket.

There was a ten minute interval while two of our players donned the umpires' coats and our openers strapped on their pads. Tom Willis showed me the batting list he had drawn up and I saw without surprise that I was last man in.

'Our team's packed with batting, Mr Herriot,' he said seriously. 'I couldn't find a place for you higher up the order.'

Mr Blenkinsopp, preparing to receive the first ball, really looked the part, gay cap pulled well down, college colours bright on the broad V of his sweater. But in this particular situation he had one big disadvantage; he was too good.

All the coaching he had received had been aimed at keeping the ball down. An 'uppish' stroke was to be deplored. But everything had to be uppish on this pitch.

As I watched from my place on the form he stepped out and executed a flawless cover drive. At Headingley the ball would have rattled against the boards for four but here it travelled approximately two and a half feet and the fat lad stooped carelessly, lifted it from the dense vegetation and threw it back to the bowler. The next one the curate picked beautifully off his toes and flicked it to square leg for what would certainly have been another four anywhere else. This one went for about a yard before the jungle claimed it.

It saddened me to watch him having to resort to swiping tactics which were clearly foreign to him. He did manage to get in a few telling blows but was caught on the boundary for twelve.

It was a bad start for Rainby with that large total facing them and the two Hedwick fast bowlers looked very formidable. One of them in particular, a gangling youth with great long arms and a shock of red hair seemed to fire his missiles with the speed of light, making the batsmen duck and dodge as the ball flew around their ears.

'That's Tagger Hird,' explained my nearest team mate on the bench. 'By gaw 'e does chuck 'em down. It's a bugger facin' him when the light's getting bad.'

I nodded in silence. I wasn't looking forward to facing him at all, in any kind of light. In fact I was dreading any further display of my shortcomings and I had the feeling that walking out there to the middle was going to be the worst part of all.

But meanwhile I couldn't help responding to the gallant fight Rainby were putting up. As the match went on I found we had some stalwarts in our ranks. Bert Chapman the council roadman and an old acquaintance of mine strode out with his ever present wide grin splitting his brick-red face and began to hoist the ball all over the field. At the other end Maurice Briggs the blacksmith, sleeves rolled high over his mighty biceps and the bat looking like a Woolworths toy in his huge hands, clouted six after six, showing a marked preference for the ravine where there now lurked some hapless member of the other team. I felt for him, whoever it was down there; the sun had gone behind the hills and the light was fading and it must have been desperately gloomy in those humid depths.

And then when Tom came in he showed the true strategical sense of a captain. When Hedwick were batting it had not escaped his notice that they aimed a lot of their shots at a broad patch of particularly impenetrable vegetation, a mato grosso of rank verdure containing not only tangled grasses but nettles, thistles and an abundance of nameless flora. The memory of the Hedwick batsmen running up and down while his fielders thrashed about in there was fresh in his mind as he batted, and at every opportunity he popped one with the greatest accuracy into the jungle himself.

It was the kind of innings you would expect from him; not spectacular, but thoughtful and methodical. After one well-placed drive he ran seventeen while the fielders clawed at the undergrowth and the yells from the wall took on a frantic note.

And all the time we were creeping nearer to the total. When eight wickets had fallen we had reached a hundred and forty and our batsmen were running whether they hit the ball or not. It was too dark by now, to see, in any case, with great black banks of cloud driving over the fell top and the beginnings of a faint drizzle in the air.

In the gathering gloom I watched as the batsman swung, but only managed to push the ball a few yards up the pitch. Nevertheless he broke into a full gallop and collided with his partner

175

who was roaring up from the other end. They fell in a heap with the ball underneath and the wicketkeeper, in an attempt at a run-out, dived among the bodies and scrabbled desperately for the ball. Animal cries broke out from the heads on the wall, the players were all bellowing at each other and at that moment I think the last of my romantic illusions about cricket slipped quietly away.

But soon I had no more time to think about such things. There was an eldritch scream from the bowler and our man was out L.B.W. It was my turn to bat.

Our score was a hundred and forty-five and as, dry-mouthed, I buckled on my pads, the lines of the poem came back to me. 'Ten to win and the last man in.' But I had never dreamed that my first innings in a cricket match would be like this, with the rain pattering steadily on the grass and the oil lamps on the farm winking through the darkness.

Pacing my way to the wicket I passed close by Tagger Hird who eyed me expressionlessly, tossing the ball from one meaty hand to another and whistling softly to himself. As I took guard he began his pounding run up and I braced myself. He had already dropped two of our batsmen in groaning heaps and I realised I had small hope of even seeing the ball.

But I had decided on one thing! I wasn't going to just stand there and take it. I wasn't a cricketer but I was going to try to hit the ball. And as Tagger arrived at full gallop and brought his arm over I stepped out and aimed a violent lunge at where I thought the thing might be. Nothing happened. I heard the smack on the sodden turf and the thud into the wicketkeeper's gloves, that was all.

The same thing happened with the next two deliveries. Great flailing blows which nearly swung me off my feet but nothing besides the smack and the thud. As Tagger ran up the fourth time I was breathless and my heart was thumping. I was playing a whirlwind innings except that I hadn't managed to make contact so far.

Again the arm came over and again I leapt out. And this time there was a sharp crack. I had got a touch but I had no idea where the ball had gone. I was standing gazing stupidly around me when I heard a bellowed '*Come on!*' and saw my partner thundering towards me. At the same time I spotted a couple of fielders running after something away down on my left and then the umpire made a signal. I had scored a four.

With the fifth ball I did the same thing and heard another crack, but this time, as I glared wildly about me I saw there was activity somewhere behind me on my right. We ran three and I had made seven.

There had been a no-ball somewhere and with the extra delivery Tagger scattered my partner's stumps and the match was over. We had lost by two runs.

'A merry knock, Mr Herriot,' Tom said, as I marched from the arena. 'Just for a minute I was beginnin' to think you were goin' to pull it off for us there.'

There was a pie and pea supper for both teams in the pub and as I settled down with a frothing pint of beer the thought kept coming back to me. Seven not out! After the humiliations of the evening it was an ultimate respectability. I had not at any time seen the ball during my innings and I had no idea how it had arrived in those two places but I had made seven not out. And as the meal arrived in front of me – delicious home-made steak and kidney pie with mounds of mushy peas – and I looked around at the roomful of laughing sunburnt men I began to feel good.

Tom sat on one side of me and Mr Blenkinsopp on the other. I had been interested to see that the curate could sink a pint with the best of them and he smiled as he put down his glass.

'Well done indeed, James. Nearly a story book ending. And you know, I'm quite sure you'd have clinched it if your partner had been able to keep going.'

I felt myself blushing. 'Well it's very kind of you, but I was a bit lucky.'

'Lucky? Not a bit of it!' said Mr Blenkinsopp. 'You played two beautiful strokes – I don't know how you did it in the conditions.'

'Beautiful strokes?'

'Most certainly. A delightful leg glance followed by a late cut of the greatest delicacy. Don't you agree, Tom?'

Tom sprinkled a little salt on his peas and turned to me, 'Ah do agree. And the best bit was how you got 'em up in the air to clear t'long grass. That was clever that was.' He conveyed a forkful of pie to his mouth and began to munch stolidly.

I looked at him narrowly. Tom was always serious so there was nothing to be learned from his expression. He was always kind, too, he had been kind all evening.

But I really think he meant it this time.

26

'Is this the thing you've been telling me about?' I asked.

Mr Wilkin nodded. 'Aye, that's it, it's always like that.'

I looked down at the helpless convulsions of the big dog lying at my feet; at the staring eyes, the wildly pedalling limbs. The farmer had told me about the periodic attacks which had begun to affect his sheepdog, Gyp, but it was coincidence that one should occur when I was on the farm for another reason.

'And he's all right afterwards, you say?'

'Right as a bobbin. Seems a bit dazed, maybe, for about an hour then he's back to normal.' The farmer shrugged. 'I've had lots o' dogs through my hands as you know and I've seen plenty of dogs with fits. I thought I knew all the causes – worms, wrong feeding, distemper – but this has me beat. I've tried everything.'

'Well you can stop trying, Mr Wilkin,' I said. 'You won't be able to do much for Gyp. He's got epilepsy.'

'Epilepsy? But he's a grand, normal dog most of t'time.'

'Yes, I know. That's how it goes. There's nothing actually wrong with his brain – it's a mysterious condition. The cause is unknown but it's almost certainly hereditary.'

Mr Wilkin raised his eyebrows. 'Well that's a rum 'un. If it's hereditary why hasn't it shown up before now ? He's nearly two years old and he didn't start this till a few weeks ago.'

'That's typical,' I replied. 'Eighteen months to two years is about the time it usually appears.'

Gyp interrupted us by getting up and staggering towards his master, wagging his tail. He seemed untroubled by his experience. In fact the whole thing had lasted less than two minutes.

Mr Wilkin bent and stroked the rough head briefly. His craggy features were set in a thoughtful cast. He was a big powerful man in his forties and now as the eyes narrowed in that face which rarely smiled he looked almost menacing. I had heard more than one man say he wouldn't like to get on the wrong side of Sep Wilkin and I could see what they meant. But he had always treated me right and since he farmed nearly a thousand acres I saw quite a lot of him.

His passion was sheepdogs. A lot of farmers liked to run dogs at the trials but Mr Wilkin was one of the top men. He bred and trained dogs which regularly won at the local events and occasionally at the national trials. And what was troubling me was that Gyp was his main hope.

He had picked out the two best pups from a litter – Gyp and Sweep – and had trained them with the dedication that had made him a winner. I don't think I have ever seen two dogs enjoy each other quite as much; whenever I was on the farm I would see them together, sometimes peeping nose by nose over the half door of the loose box where they slept, occasionally slinking devotedly round the feet of their master but usually just playing together. They must have spent hours rolling about in ecstatic wrestling matches, growling and panting, gnawing gently at each other's limbs.

A few months ago George Crossley, one of Mr Wilkin's oldest friends and a keen trial man, had lost his best dog with nephritis and Mr Wilkin had let him have Sweep. I was surprised at the time because Sweep was shaping better than Gyp in his training and looked like turning out a real champion. But it was Gyp who remained. He must have missed his friend but there were other dogs on the farm and if they didn't quite make up for Sweep he was never really lonely.

As I watched, I could see the dog recovering rapidly. It was extraordinary how soon normality was restored after that frightening convulsion. And I waited with some apprehension to hear what his master would say.

The cold, logical decision for him to make would be to have Gyp put down and, looking at the friendly, tail-wagging animal I didn't like the idea at all. There was something very attractive about him. The big-boned, well-marked body was handsome but his most distinctive feature was his head where one ear somehow contrived to stick up while the other lay flat, giving him a lop-sided, comic appeal. Gyp, in fact, looked a bit of a clown. But a clown who radiated goodwill and camaraderie.

Mr Wilkin spoke at last. 'Will he get any better as he grows older?'

'Almost certainly not,' I replied.

'Then he'll always 'ave these fits?'

'I'm afraid so. You say he has them every two or three weeks – well it will probably carry on more or less like that with occasional variations.'

'But he could have one any time?'

'Yes.'

'In the middle of a trial, like.' The farmer sunk his head on his chest and his voice rumbled deep. 'That's it, then.'

In the long silence which followed, the fateful words became more and more inevitable. Sep Wilkin wasn't the man to hesitate in a matter which concerned his ruling passion. Ruthless culling of any animal which didn't come up to standard would be his policy. When he finally cleared his throat I had a sinking premonition of what he was going to say.

But I was wrong.

'If I kept him, could you do anything for him?' he asked.

'Well I could give you some pills for him. They might decrease the frequency of the fits.' I tried to keep the eagerness out of my voice.

'Right . . . right . . . I'll come into t'surgery and get some,' he muttered.

'Fine. But . . . er . . . you won't ever breed from him, will you you?' I said.

'Naw, naw, naw,' the farmer grunted with a touch of irritability as though he didn't want to pursue the matter further.

And I held my peace because I felt intuitively that he did not want to be detected in a weakness; that he was prepared to keep the dog simply as a pet. It was funny how events began to slot into place and suddenly make sense. That was why he had let Sweep, the superior trial dog, go. He just liked Gyp. In fact Sep Wilkin, hard man though he may be, had succumbed to that off-beat charm.

So I shifted to some light chatter about the weather as I walked back to the car, but when I was about to drive off the farmer returned to the main subject.

'There's one thing about Gyp I never mentioned,' he said, bending to the window. 'I don't know whether it has owt to do with the job or not. He has never barked in his life.'

I looked at him in surprise. 'You mean never, ever?'

'That's right. Not a single bark. T'other dogs make a noise when strangers come on the farm but I've never heard Gyp utter a sound since he was born.'

'Well that's very strange,' I said. 'But I can't see that it is connected with his condition in any way.'

And as I switched on the engine I noticed for the first time that while a bitch and two half grown pups gave tongue to see me on my way Gyp merely regarded me in his comradely way, mouth open, tongue lolling, but made no noise. A silent dog.

The thing intrigued me. So much so that whenever I was on the farm over the next few months I made a point of watching the big sheepdog at whatever he was doing. But there was never any change. Between the convulsions which had settled down to around three week intervals he was a normal active happy animal. But soundless.

I saw him, too, in Darrowby when his master came in to market. Gyp was often seated comfortably in the back of the car, but if I happened to speak to Mr Wilkin on these occasions I kept off the subject because, as I said, I had the feeling that he more than most farmers would hate to be exposed in keeping a dog for other than working purposes.

And yet I have always entertained a suspicion that most farm dogs were more or less pets. The dogs on sheep farms were of course indispensable working animals and on other establishments they no doubt performed a function in helping to bring in the cows. But watching them on my daily rounds I often wondered. I saw them rocking along on carts at haytime, chasing rats among the stooks at harvest, pottering around the buildings or roaming the fields at the side of the farmer; and I wondered . . . what did they really do?

My suspicions were strengthened at other times – as when I was trying to round up some cattle into a corner and the dog tried to get into the act by nipping at a hock or tail. There was invariably a hoarse yell of 'Siddown, dog!' or 'Gerrout, dog!'

So right up to the present day I still stick to my theory; most farm dogs are pets and they are there mainly because the farmer just likes to have them around. You would have to put a farmer on the rack to get him to admit it but I think I am right. And in the process those dogs have a wonderful time. They don't have to beg for walks, they are out all day long, and in the company of their masters. If I want to find a man on a farm I look for his dog, knowing the man won't be far away. I try to give my own dogs a good life but it cannot compare with the life of the average farm dog.

There was a long spell when Sep Wilkin's stock stayed healthy and I didn't see either him or Gyp, then I came across them both by accident at a sheepdog trial. It was a local event run in conjunction with the Mellerton Agricultural Show and since I was in the district I decided to steal an hour off.

I took Helen with me, too, because these trials have always fascinated us. The wonderful control of the owners over their animals, the intense involvement of the dogs themselves, the sheer skill of the whole operation always held us spellbound.

She put her arm through mine as we went in at the entrance gate to where a crescent of cars was drawn up at one end of a long field. The field was on the river's edge and through a fringe of trees the afternoon sunshine glinted on the tumbling water of the shallows and turned the long beach of bleached stones to a dazzling white. Groups of men, mainly competitors, stood around chatting as they watched. They were quiet, easy, bronzed men and as they seemed to be drawn from all social strata from prosperous farmers to working men their garb was varied; cloth caps, trilbies, deerstalkers or no hat at all; tweed jackets, stiff best suits, open-necked shirts, fancy ties, sometimes neither collar nor tie. Nearly all of them leaned on long crooks with the handles fashioned from rams' horns.

Snatches of talk reached us as we walked among them.

'You got 'ere, then, Fred.' 'That's a good gather.' 'Nay, 'e's missed one, 'e'll get nowt for that.' 'Them sheep's a bit flighty.' 'Aye they're buggers.' And above it all the whistles of the man running a dog; every conceivable level and pitch of whistle with now and then a shout. 'Sit!' 'Get by!' Every man had his own way with his dog.

The dogs waiting their turn were tied up to a fence with a hedge growing over it. There were about seventy of them and it was rather wonderful to see that long row of waving tails and friendly expressions. They were mostly strangers to each other but there wasn't even the semblance of disagreement, never mind a fight. It seemed that the natural obedience of these little creatures was linked to an amicable disposition.

This appeared to be common to their owners, too. There was no animosity, no resentment at defeat, no unseemly display of triumph in victory. If a man overran his time he ushered his group of sheep quietly in the corner and returned with a philosophical grin to his colleagues. There was a little quiet leg-pulling but that was all.

We came across Sep Wilkin leaning against his car at the best vantage point about thirty yards away from the final pen. Gyp, tied to the bumper, turned and gave me his crooked grin while

Mrs Wilkin on a camp stool by his side rested a hand on his shoulder. Gyp, it seemed, had got under her skin too.

Helen went over to speak to her and I turned to her husband. 'Are you running a dog today, Mr Wilkin?'

'No, not this time, just come to watch. I know a lot o' the dogs.'

I stood near him for a while watching the competitors in action, breathing in the clean smell of trampled grass and plug tobacco. In front of us next to the pen the judge stood by his post.

I had been there for about ten minutes when Mr Wilkin lifted a pointing finger. 'Look who's there!'

George Crossley with Sweep trotting at his heels was making his way unhurriedly to the post. Gyp suddenly stiffened and sat up very straight, his cocked ears accentuating the lop-sided look. It was many months since he had seen his brother and companion; it seemed unlikely I thought, that he would remember him. But his interest was clearly intense, and as the judge waved his white handkerchief and the three sheep were released from the far corner he rose slowly to his feet.

A gesture from Mr Crossley sent Sweep winging round the perimeter of the field in a wide, joyous gallop and as he neared the sheep a whistle dropped him on his belly. From then on it was an object lesson in the cooperation of man and dog. Sep Wilkin had always said Sweep would be a champion and he looked the part, darting and falling at his master's commands. Short piercing whistles, shrill plaintive whistles; he was in tune with them all.

No dog all day had brought his sheep through the three lots of gates as effortlessly as Sweep did now and as he approached the pen near us it was obvious that he would win the cup unless some disaster struck. But this was the touchy bit; more than once with other dogs the sheep had broken free and gone bounding away within feet of the wooden rails.

George Crossley held the gate wide and extended his crook. You could see now why they all carried those long sticks. His commands to Sweep, huddled flat along the turf, were now almost inaudible but the quiet words brought the dog inching first one way then the other. The sheep were in the entrance to the pen now but they still looked around them irresolutely and the game was not over yet. But as Sweep wriggled towards them almost imperceptibly they turned and entered and Mr Crossley crashed the gate behind them.

As he did so he turned to Sweep with a happy cry of '*Good lad!*' and the dog responded with a quick jerking wag of his tail.

At that, Gyp, who had been standing very tall, watching every move with the most intense concentration raised his head and emitted a single resounding bark.

'*Woof!*' went Gyp as we all stared at him in astonishment.

'Did you hear that?' gasped Mrs Wilkin.

'Well, by gaw!' her husband burst out, looking open-mouthed at his dog.

Gyp didn't seem to be aware that he had done anything unusual. He was too preoccupied by the reunion with his brother and within seconds the two dogs were rolling around, chewing playfully at each other as of old.

I suppose the Wilkins as well as myself had the feeling that this event might start Gyp barking like any other dog, but it was not to be.

Six years later I was on the farm and went to the house to get some hot water. As Mrs Wilkin handed me the bucket she looked down at Gyp who was basking in the sunshine outside the kitchen window.

'There you are, then, funny fellow,' she said to the dog.

I laughed. 'Has he ever barked since that day?'

Mrs Wilkin shook her head. 'No he hasn't, not a sound. I waited a long time but I know he's not going to do it now.'

'Ah well, it's not important. But still, I'll never forget that afternoon at the trial,' I said.

'Nor will I!' She looked at Gyp again and her eyes softened in reminiscence. 'Poor old lad, eight years old and only one woof!'

27

A full surgery! But the ripple of satisfaction as I surveyed the packed rows of heads waned quickly as realisation dawned. It was only the Dimmocks again.

I first encountered the Dimmocks one evening when I had a call to a dog which had been knocked down by a car. The address was down in the old part of the town and I was cruising slowly along the row of decaying cottages looking for the number when a door burst open and three shock-headed little children ran into the street and waved me down frantically.

'He's in 'ere, Mister!' they gasped in unison as I got out, and then began immediately to put me in the picture.

'It's Bonzo!' 'Aye, a car 'it 'im!' 'We 'ad to carry 'im in, Mister!' They all got their words in as I opened the garden gate and struggled up the path with the three of them hanging on to my arms and tugging at my coat; and en route I gazed in wonder at the window of the house where a mass of other young faces mouthed at me and a tangle of arms gesticulated.

Once through the door which opened directly into the living room I was swamped by a rush of bodies and borne over to the corner where I saw my patient.

Bonzo was sitting upright on a ragged blanket. He was a large shaggy animal of indeterminate breed and though at a glance there didn't seem to be much ailing him he wore a pathetic expression of self pity. Since everybody was talking at once I decided to ignore them and carry out my examination. I worked my way over legs, pelvis, ribs and spine; no fractures. His mucous membranes were a good colour, there was no evidence of internal injury. In fact the only thing I could find was slight bruising over the left shoulder. Bonzo had sat like a statue as I felt over him, but as I finished he toppled over on to his side and lay looking up at me apologetically, his tail thumping on the blanket.

'You're a big soft dog, that's what you are,' I said and the tail thumped faster.

I turned and viewed the throng and after a moment or two managed to pick out the parents. Mum was fighting her way to the front while at the rear, Dad, a diminutive figure, was beaming at me over the heads. I did a bit of shushing and when the babel died down I addressed myself to Mrs Dimmock.

'I think he's been lucky,' I said. 'I can't find any serious injury. I think the car must have bowled him over and knocked the wind out of him for a minute, or he may have been suffering from shock.'

The uproar broke out again. 'Will 'e die, Mister?' 'What's the matter with 'im?' 'What are you going to do?'

I gave Bonzo an injection of a mild sedative while he lay rigid, a picture of canine suffering, with the tousled heads looking down at him with deep concern and innumerable little hands poking out and caressing him.

Mrs Dimmock produced a basin of hot water and while I washed my hands I was able to make a rough assessment of the household. I counted eleven little Dimmocks from a boy in his early teens down to a grubby faced infant crawling around the floor; and judging by the significant bulge in Mum's midriff the number was soon to be augmented. They were clad in a motley selection of hand-me-downs; darned pullovers, patched trousers, tattered dresses, yet the general atmosphere in the house was of unconfined *joie de vivre*.

Bonzo wasn't the only animal and I stared in disbelief as another biggish dog and a cat with two half grown kittens appeared from among the crowding legs and feet. I would have thought that the problem of filling the human mouths would have been difficult enough without importing several animals.

But the Dimmocks didn't worry about such things; they did what they wanted to do, and they got by. Dad, I learned later, had never done any work within living memory. He had a 'bad back' and lived what seemed to me a reasonably gracious life, roaming interestedly around the town by day and enjoying a

187

quiet beer and a game of dominoes in a corner of the Four Horse Shoes by night.

I saw him quite often; he was easy to pick out because he invariably carried a walking stick which gave him an air of dignity and he always walked briskly and purposefully as though he were going somewhere important.

I took a final look at Bonzo, still stretched on the blanket, looking up at me with soulful eyes then I struggled towards the door.

'I don't think there's anything to worry about,' I shouted above the chattering which had speedily broken out again, 'but I'll look in tomorrow and make sure.'

When I drew up outside the house next morning I could see Bonzo lolloping around the garden with several of the children. They were passing a ball from one to the other and he was leaping ecstatically high in the air to try to intercept it.

He was clearly none the worse for his accident but when he saw me opening the gate his tail went down and he dropped almost to his knees and slunk into the house. The children received me rapturously.

'You've made 'im better, Mister!' 'He's all right now, isn't he?' 'He's 'ad a right big breakfast this mornin', Mister!'

I went inside with little hands clutching at my coat. Bonzo was sitting bolt upright on his blanket in the same attitude as the previous evening, but as I approached he slowly collapsed on to his side and lay looking up at me with a martyred expression.

I laughed as I knelt by him. 'You're the original old soldier, Bonzo, but you can't fool me. I saw you out there.'

I gently touched the bruised shoulder and the big dog tremblingly closed his eyes as he resigned himself to his fate. Then when I stood up and he realised he wasn't going to have another injection he leapt to his feet and bounded away into the garden.

There was a chorus of delighted cries from the Dimmocks and they turned and looked at me with undisguised admiration. Clearly they considered that I had plucked Bonzo from the jaws of death. Mr Dimmock stepped forward from the mass.

'You'll send me a bill, won't you,' he said, with the dignity that was peculiar to him.

My first glance last night had decided me that this was a no-charging job and I hadn't even written it in the book, but I nodded solemnly.

'Very well, Mr Dimmock, I'll do that.'

And throughout our long association, though no money ever changed hands, he always said the same thing – 'You'll send me a bill, won't you.'

This was the beginning of my close relationship with the Dimmocks. Obviously they had taken a fancy to me and wanted to see as much as possible of me. Over the succeeding weeks and months they brought in a varied selection of dogs, cats, budgies, rabbits at frequent intervals, and when they found that my services were free they stepped up the number of visits; and when one came they all came. I was anxiously trying to expand the small animal side of the practice and increasingly my hopes were raised momentarily then dashed when I opened the door and saw a packed waiting room.

And it increased the congestion when they started bringing their auntie, Mrs Pounder, from down the road with them to see what a nice chap I was. Mrs Pounder, a fat lady who always wore a greasy velour hat perched on an untidy mound of hair, evidently shared the family tendency to fertility and usually brought a few of her own ample brood with her.

That is how it was this particular morning. I swept the assembled company with my eye but could discern only beaming Dimmocks and Pounders; and this time I couldn't even pick out my patient. Then the assembly parted and spread out as though by prearranged signal and I saw little Nellie Dimmock with a tiny puppy on her knee.

Nellie was my favourite. Mind you, I liked all the family; in fact they were such nice people that I always enjoyed their visits after that first disappointment. Mum and Dad were always courteous and cheerful and the children, though boisterous, were never ill-mannered; they were happy and friendly and if

189

they saw me in the street they would wave madly and go on waving till I was out of sight. And I saw them often because they were continually scurrying around the town doing odd jobs – delivering milk or papers. Best of all, they loved their animals and were kind to them.

But as I say, Nellie was my favourite. She was about nine and had suffered an attack of 'infantile paralysis', as it used to be called, when very young. It had left her with a pronounced limp and a frailty which set her apart from her robust brothers and sisters. Her painfully thin legs seemed almost too fragile to carry her around but above the pinched face her hair, the colour of ripe corn, flowed to her shoulders and her eyes, though slightly crossed, gazed out calm and limpid blue through steel-rimmed spectacles.

'What's that you've got, Nellie?' I asked.

'It's a little dog,' she almost whispered. ''e's mine.'

'You mean he's your very own?'

She nodded proudly. 'Aye, 'e's mine.'

'He doesn't belong to your brothers and sisters, too?'

'Naw, 'e's mine.'

Rows of Dimmock and Pounder heads nodded in eager acquiescence as Nellie lifted the puppy to her cheek and looked up at me with a smile of a strange sweetness. It was a smile that always tugged at my heart; full of a child's artless happiness and trust but with something else which was poignant and maybe had to do with the way Nellie was.

'Well, he looks a fine dog to me,' I said. 'He's a Spaniel, isn't he?'

She ran a hand over the little head. 'Aye, a Cocker. Mr Brown said 'e was a Cocker.'

There was a slight disturbance at the back and Mr Dimmock appeared from the crush. He gave a respectful cough.

'He's a proper pure bred, Mr Herriot,' he said. 'Mr Brown from the bank's bitch had a litter and 'e gave this 'un to Nellie.' He tucked his stick under his arm and pulled a long envelope from an inside pocket. He handed it to me with a flourish. 'That's 'is pedigree.'

I read it through and whistled softly. 'He's a real blue-blooded hound, all right, and I see he's got a big long name. Darrowby Tobias the third. My word, that sounds great.'

I looked down at the little girl again. 'And what do *you* call him, Nellie?'

'Toby,' she said softly. 'I calls 'im Toby.'

I laughed. 'All right, then. What's the matter with Toby anyway. Why have you brought him?'

'He's been sick, Mr Herriot.' Mrs Dimmock spoke from somewhere among the heads. 'He can't keep nothin' down.'

'Well I know what that'll be. Has he been wormed?'

'No, don't think so.'

'I should think he just needs a pill,' I said. 'But bring him through and I'll have a look at him.'

Other clients were usually content to send one representative through with their animals but the Dimmocks all had to come. I marched along with the crowd behind me filling the passage from wall to wall. Our consulting-cum-operating room was quite small and I watched with some apprehension as the procession filed in after me. But they all got in, Mrs Pounder, her velour hat slightly askew, squeezing herself in with some difficulty at the rear.

My examination of the puppy took longer than usual as I had to fight my way to the thermometer on the trolley then struggle in the other direction to get the stethoscope from its hook on the wall. But I finished at last.

'Well I can't find anything wrong with him,' I said. 'So I'm pretty sure he just has a tummy full of worms. I'll give you a pill now and you must give it to him first thing tomorrow morning.'

Like a football match turning out, the mass of people surged along the passage and into the street and another Dimmock visit had come to an end.

I forgot the incident immediately because there was nothing unusual about it. The pot-bellied appearance of the puppy made my diagnosis a formality; I didn't expect to see him again.

But I was wrong. A week later my surgery was once more overflowing and I had another squashed-in session with Toby in the little back room. My pill had evacuated a few worms but he was still vomiting, still distended.

'Are you giving him five very small meals a day as I told you?' I asked.

I received emphatic affirmative and I believed them. The Dimmocks really took care of their animals. There was something else here, yet I couldn't find it. Temperature normal, lungs clear, abdomen negative on palpation; I couldn't make it out. I dispensed a bottle of our antacid mixture with a feeling of defeat. A young puppy like this shouldn't need such a thing.

This was the beginning of a frustrating period. There would be a span of two or three weeks when I would think the trouble had righted itself then without warning the place would be full of Dimmocks and Pounders and I'd be back where I started.

And all the time Toby was growing thinner.

I tried everything; gastric sedatives, variations of diet, quack remedies. I interrogated the Dimmocks repeatedly about the character of the vomiting – how long after eating, what were the intervals between, and I received varying replies. Sometimes he brought his food straight back, at others he retained it for several hours. I got nowhere.

It must have been over eight weeks later – Toby would be about four months old – when I again viewed the assembled Dimmocks with a sinking heart. Their visits had become depressing affairs and I could not foresee anything better today as I opened the waiting-room door and allowed myself to be almost carried along the passage. This time it was Dad who was the last to wedge himself into the consulting room then Nellie placed the little dog on the table.

I felt an inward lurch of sheer misery. Toby had grown despite his disability and was now a grim caricature of a Cocker Spaniel, the long silky ears drooping from an almost fleshless skull, the spindly legs pathetically feathered. I had thought Nellie was thin but her pet had outdone her. And he wasn't just thin, he was trembling slightly as he stood arch-backed on the smooth surface, and his face had the dull inward look of an animal which has lost interest.

The little girl ran her hand along the jutting ribs and the pale, squinting eyes looked up at me through the steel spectacles with that smile which pulled at me more painfully than ever before. She didn't seem worried. Probably she had no idea how things were, but whether she had or not I knew I'd never be able to tell her that her dog was slowly dying.

I rubbed my eyes wearily. 'What has he had to eat today?'

Nellie answered herself. 'He's 'ad some bread and milk.'

'How long ago was that?' I asked, but before anybody could reply the little dog vomited, sending the half digested stomach contents soaring in a graceful arc to land two feet away on the table.

I swung round on Mrs Dimmock. 'Does he always do it like that?'

'Aye he mostly does – sends it flying out, like.'

'But why didn't you tell me?'

The poor lady looked flustered. 'Well ... I don't know ... I ...'

I held up a hand. 'That's all right, Mrs Dimmock, never mind.' It occurred to me that all the way through my totally ineffectual treatment of this dog not a single Dimmock or Pounder had uttered a word of criticism so why should I start to complain now?

But I knew what Toby's trouble was now. At last, at long last I knew.

And in case my present day colleagues reading this may think I had been more than usually thick-headed in my handling of the case I would like to offer in my defence that such limited text books as there were in those days made only a cursory reference to pyloric stenosis (narrowing of the exit of the stomach where it joins the small intestine) and if they did they said nothing about treatment.

But surely, I thought, somebody in England was ahead of the books. There must be people who were actually doing this operation ... and if there were I had a feeling one might not be too far away ...

I worked my way through the crush and trotted along the

passage to the phone.

'Is that you, Granville?'

'*Jim!*' A bellow of pure unalloyed joy. 'How are you, laddie?'

'Very well, how are you?'

'Ab-so-lutely tip top, old son! Never better!'

'Granville, I've got a four-month-old spaniel pup I'd like to bring through to you. It's got pyloric stenosis.'

'Oh lovely!'

'I'm afraid the little thing's just about on its last legs – a bag of bones.'

'Splendid, splendid!'

'This is because I've been mucking about for four weeks in ignorance.'

'Fine, just fine!'

'And the owners are a very poor family. They can't pay anything I'm afraid.'

'Wonderful!'

I hesitated a moment. 'Granville, you do ... er ... you have ... operated on these cases before?'

'Did five yesterday.'

'What!'

A deep rumble of laughter. 'I do but jest, old son, but you needn't worry, I've done a few. And it isn't such a bad job.'

'Well that's great.' I looked at my watch. 'It's half past nine now, I'll get Siegfried to take over my morning round and I'll see you before eleven.'

28

Granville had been called out when I arrived and I hung around his surgery till I heard the expensive sound of the Bentley purring into the yard. Through the window I saw yet another magnificent pipe glinting behind the wheel then my colleague, in an impeccable pin-striped suit which made him look like the Director of the Bank of England, paced majestically towards the side door.

'Good to see you, Jim!' he exclaimed, wringing my hand warmly. Then before removing his jacket he took his pipe from his mouth and regarded it with a trace of anxiety for a second before giving it a polish with his yellow cloth and placing it tenderly in a drawer.

It wasn't long before I was under the lamp in the operating room bending over Toby's small outstretched form while Granville – the other Granville Bennett – worked with fierce concentration inside the abdomen of the little animal.

'You see the gross gastric dilatation,' he murmured. 'Classical lesion.' He gripped the pylorus and poised his scalpel. 'Now I'm going through the serous coat.' A quick deft incision. 'A bit of blunt dissection here for the muscle fibres ... down ... down ... a little more ... ah, there it is, can you see it – the mucosa bulging into the cleft. Yes ... yes ... just right. That's what you've got to arrive at.'

I peered down at the tiny tube which had been the site of all Toby's troubles. 'Is that all, then?'

'That's all, laddie.' He stepped back with a grin. 'The obstruction is relieved now and you can take bets that this little chap will start to put weight on now.'

'That's wonderful, Granville. I'm really grateful.'

'Nonsense, Jim, it was a pleasure. You can do the next one yourself now, eh?' He laughed, seized needle and sutures and sewed up the abdominal muscles and skin at an impossible pace.

A few minutes later he was in his office pulling on his jacket, then as he filled his pipe he turned to me.

'I've got a little plan for the rest of the morning, laddie.'

I shrank away from him and threw up a protective hand. 'Well now, er ... it's kind of you, Granville, but I really ... I honestly must get back ... we're very busy, you know ... can't leave Siegfried too long . . . work'll be piling up . . .' I stopped because I felt I was beginning to gibber.

My colleague looked wounded. 'All I meant, old son, was that we want you to come to lunch. Zoe is expecting you.'

'Oh . . . oh, I see. Well that's very kind. We're not going . . . anywhere else, then?'

'Anywhere else?' He blew out his cheeks and spread his arms wide. 'Of course not. I just have to call in at my branch surgery on the way.'

'Branch surgery? I didn't know you had one.'

'Oh yes, just a stone's throw from my house.' He put an arm round my shoulders. 'Well let's go, shall we?'

As I lay back, cradled in the Bentley's luxury, I dwelt happily on the thought that at last I was going to meet Zoe Bennett when I was my normal self. She would learn this time that I wasn't a perpetually drunken oaf. In fact the next hour or two seemed full of rosy promise; an excellent lunch illumined by my witty conversation and polished manners, then back with Toby, magically resuscitated, to Darrowby.

I smiled to myself when I thought of Nellie's face when I told her her pet was going to be able to eat and grow strong and play-ful like any other pup. I was still smiling when the car pulled up on the outskirts of Granville's home village. I glanced idly through the window at a low stone building with leaded panes and a wooden sign dangling over the entrance. It read 'Old Oak Tree Inn'. I turned quickly to my companion.

'I thought we were going to your branch surgery?'

Granville gave me a smile of childish innocence. 'Oh that's what I call this place. It's so near home and I transact quite a lot of business here.' He patted my knee. 'We'll just pop in for an appetiser, eh?'

'Now wait a minute,' I stammered, gripping the sides of my seat tightly. 'I just can't be late today. I'd much rather . . .'

Granville raised a hand. 'Jim, laddie, we won't be in for long.' He looked at his watch. 'It's exactly twelve thirty and I promised Zoe we'd be home by one o'clock. She's cooking roast beef and Yorkshire pudding and it would take a braver man than me to let her pudding go flat. I guarantee we'll be in that house at one o'clock on the dot – O.K. ?'

I hesitated. I couldn't come to much harm in half an hour. I climbed out of the car.

As we went into the pub a large man, who had been leaning on the counter, turned and exchanged enthusiastic greetings with my colleague.

'Albert!' cried Granville. 'Meet Jim Herriot from Darrowby. Jim, this is Albert Wainright, the landlord of the Wagon and Horses over in Matherley. In fact he's the president of the Licensed Victuallers' Association this year, aren't you, Albert ?'

The big man grinned and nodded and for a moment I felt overwhelmed by the two figures on either side of me. It was difficult to describe the hard, bulky tissue of Granville's construction but Mr Wainright was unequivocally fat. A checked jacket hung open to display an enormous expanse of striped shirted abdomen overflowing the waistband of his trousers. Above a gay bow tie cheerful eyes twinkled at me from a red face and when he spoke his tone was rich and fruity. He embodied the rich ambience of the term 'Licensed Victualler'.

I began to sip the half pint of beer I had ordered but when another appeared in two minutes I saw I was going to fall hopelessly behind and switched to the whiskies and sodas which the others were drinking. And my undoing was that both my companions appeared to have a standing account here; they downed their drinks, tapped softly on the counter and said, 'Yes please, Jack,' whereupon three more glasses appeared with magical speed. I never had a chance to buy a round. In fact no money ever changed hands.

It was a quiet, friendly little session with Albert and Granville carrying on a conversation of the utmost good humour punctuated by the almost soundless taps on the bar. And as I fought to keep up with the two virtuosos the taps came more and more frequently till I seemed to hear them every few seconds.

Granville was as good as his word. When it was nearly one o'clock he looked at his watch.

'Got to be off now, Albert. Zoe's expecting us right now.'

And as the car rolled to a stop outside the house dead on time I realised with a dull despair that it had happened to me again. Within me a witch's brew was beginning to bubble, sending choking fumes into my brain. I felt terrible and I knew for sure I would get rapidly worse.

Granville, fresh and debonair as ever, leaped out and led me into the house.

'Zoe, my love!' he warbled, embracing his wife as she came through from the kitchen.

When she disengaged herself she came over to me. She was wearing a flowered apron which made her look if possible even more attractive.

'Hel-*lo*!' she cried and gave me that look which she shared with her husband as though meeting James Herriot was an unbelievable boon. 'Lovely to see you again. I'll get lunch now.' I replied with a foolish grin and she skipped away.

Flopping into an armchair I listened to Granville pouring steadily over at the sideboard. He put a glass in my hand and sat in another chair. Immediately the obese Staffordshire Terrier bounded on to his lap.

'Phoebles, my little pet!' he sang joyfully. 'Daddykins is home again.' And he pointed playfully at the tiny Yorkie who was who was sitting at his feet, baring her teeth repeatedly in a series of ecstatic smiles. 'And I see you, my little Victoria, I see you!'

By the time I was ushered to the table I was like a man in a dream, moving sluggishly, speaking with slurred deliberation. Granville poised himself over a vast sirloin, stropped his knife briskly then began to hack away ruthlessly. He was a prodigal server and piled about two pounds of meat on my plate then he started on the Yorkshire puddings. Instead of a single big one, Zoe had made a large number of little round ones as the farmers' wives often did, delicious golden cups, crisply brown round the sides. Granville heaped about six of these by the side of the meat as I watched stupidly. Then Zoe passed me the gravy boat.

With an effort I took a careful grip on the handle, closed one eye and began to pour. For some reason I felt I had to fill up each of the little puddings with gravy and owlishly directed the stream into one then another till they were all overflowing. Once I missed and spilled a few drops of the fragrant liquid on the tablecloth. I looked up guiltily at Zoe and giggled.

Zoe giggled back, and I had the impression that she felt that though I was a peculiar individual there was no harm in me. I just had this terrible weakness that I was never sober day or night, but I wasn't such a bad fellow at heart.

It usually took me a few days to recover from a visit to Granville and by the following Saturday I was convalescing nicely. It happened that I was in the market place and saw a large concourse of people crossing the cobbles. At first I thought from the mixture of children and adults that it must be a school outing but on closer inspection I realised it was only the Dimmocks and Pounders going shopping.

When they saw me they diverted their course and I was engulfed by a human wave.

'Look at 'im now, Mister!' 'He's eatin' like a 'oss now!' 'He's goin' to get fat soon, Mister!' The delighted cries rang around me.

Nellie had Toby on a lead and as I bent over the little animal I could hardly believe how a few days had altered him. He was still skinny but the hopeless look had gone; he was perky, ready to play. It was just a matter of time now.

His little mistress ran her hand again and again over the smooth brown coat.

'You are proud of your little dog, aren't you Nellie,' I said, and the gentle squinting eyes turned on me.

'Yes, I am.' She smiled that smile again. 'Because 'e's mine.'

29

There is plenty of time for thinking during the long hours of driving and now as I headed home from a late call my mind was idly assessing my abilities as a planner.

I had to admit that planning was not one of my strong points. Shortly after we were married I told Helen that I didn't think we should have children just at present. I pointed out that I would soon be going away, we did not have a proper home, our financial state was precarious and it would be far better to wait till after the war.

I had propounded my opinions weightily, sitting back in my chair and puffing my pipe like a sage, but I don't think I was really surprised when Helen's pregnancy was positively confirmed.

From the warm darkness the grass smell of the Dales stole through the open window and as I drove through a silent village it was mingled briefly with the mysterious sweetness of wood smoke. Beyond the houses the road curved smooth and empty between the black enclosing fells. No ... I hadn't organised things very well. Leaving Darrowby and maybe England for an indefinite period, no home, no money and a pregnant wife. It was an untidy situation. But I was beginning to realise that life was not a tidy little parcel at any time.

The clock tower showed 11 p.m. as I rolled through the market place and, turning into Trengate, I saw that the light had been turned off in our room. Helen had gone to bed. I drove round to the yard at the back, put away the car and walked down the long garden. It was the end to every day, this walk; sometimes stumbling over frozen snow but tonight moving easily through the summer darkness under the branches of the apple trees to where the house stood tall and silent against the stars.

In the passage I almost bumped into Siegfried.

'Just getting back from Allenby's, James?' he asked. 'I saw on the book that you had a colic.'

I nodded. 'Yes, but it wasn't a bad one. Just a bit of spasm. Their grey horse had been feasting on some of the hard pears lying around the orchard.'

Siegfried laughed. 'Well I've just beaten you in by a few minutes. I've been round at old Mrs Dewar's for the last hour holding her cat's paw while it had kittens.'

We reached the corner of the passage and he hesitated. 'Care for a nightcap, James?'

'I would, thanks,' I replied, and we went into the sitting room. But there was a constraint between us because Siegfried was off to London early next morning to enter the Air Force – he'd be gone before I got up – and we both knew that this was a farewell drink.

I dropped into my usual armchair while Siegfried reached into the glass-fronted cupboard above the mantelpiece and fished out the whisky bottle and glasses. He carelessly tipped out two prodigal measures and sat down opposite.

We had done a lot of this over the years, often yarning till dawn, but naturally enough it had faded since my marriage. It was like turning back the clock to sip the whisky and look at him on the other side of the fireplace and to feel, as though it were a living presence, the charm of the beautiful room with its high ceiling, graceful alcoves and french window.

We didn't talk about his departure but about the things we had always talked about and still do; the miraculous recovery of that cow, what old Mr Jenks said yesterday, the patient that knocked us flat, leapt the fence and disappeared for good. Then Siegfried raised a finger.

'Oh, James, I nearly forgot. I was tidying up the books and I find I owe you some money.'

'You do?'

'Yes, and I feel rather bad about it. It goes back to your pre-partnership days when you used to get a cut from Ewan Ross's testing. There was a slip-up somewhere and you were underpaid. Anyway, you've got fifty pounds to come.'

'Fifty pounds! Are you sure?'

'Quite sure, James, and I do apologise.'

'No need to apologise, Siegfried. It'll come in very handy right now.'

'Good, good ... anyway, the cheque's in the top drawer of the desk if you'll have a look tomorrow.' He waved a languid hand and started to talk about some sheep he had seen that afternoon.

But for a few minutes I hardly heard him. Fifty pounds! It was a lot of money in those days, especially when I would soon be earning three shillings a day as an A.C.2 during my initial training. It didn't solve my financial problem but it would be a nice little cushion to fall back on.

My nearest and dearest are pretty unanimous that I am a bit slow on the uptake and maybe they are right because it was many years later before it got through to me that there never was any fifty pounds owing. Siegfried knew I needed a bit of help at that time and when it all became clear long afterwards I realised that this was exactly how he would do it. No embarrassment to me. He hadn't even handed me the cheque. . . .

As the level in the bottle went down the conversation became more and more effortless. At one point some hours later my mind seemed to have taken on an uncanny clarity and it was as if I was disembodied and looking down at the pair of us. We had slid very low in our chairs, our heads well down the backs, legs extended far across the rug. My partner's face seemed to stand out in relief and it struck me that though he was only in his early thirties he looked a lot older. It was an attractive face, lean, strong-boned with steady humorous eyes, but not young. In fact, Siegfried, in the time I had known him, had never looked young, but he has the last laugh now because he has hardly altered with the years and is one of those who will never look old.

At that moment of the night when everything was warm and easy and I felt omniscient it seemed a pity that Tristan wasn't there to make up the familiar threesome. As we talked, the memories marched through the room like a strip of bright pictures; of November days on the hillsides with the icy rain driving into our faces, of digging the cars out of snow drifts, of the spring sunshine warming the hard countryside. And the thought recurred that Tristan had been part of it all and that I was going to miss him as much as I would miss his brother.

I could hardly believe it when Siegfried rose, threw back the curtains, and the grey light of morning streamed in. I got up and stood beside him as he looked at his watch.

'Five o'clock, James,' he said, and smiled. 'We've done it again.'

He opened the french window and we stepped into the hushed stillness of the garden. I was taking grateful gulps of the sweet air when a single bird call broke the silence.

'Did you hear that blackbird?' I said.

He nodded and I wondered if he was thinking the same thing as myself; that it sounded just like the same blackbird which had greeted the early daylight when we talked over my first case those years ago.

We went up the stairs together in silence. Siegfried stopped at his door.

'Well, James . . .' he held out his hand and his mouth twitched up at the corner.

I gripped the hand for a moment then he turned and went into his room. And as I trailed dumbly up the next flight it seemed strange that we had never said goodbye. We didn't know when, if ever, we would see each other again yet neither of us said a word. I don't know if Siegfried wanted to say anything but there was a lot trying to burst from me.

I wanted to thank him for being a friend as well as a boss, for teaching me so much, for never letting me down. There were other things, too, but I never said them.

Come to think of it, I've never even thanked him for that fifty pounds . . . until now.

30

'Look, Jim,' Helen said, 'this is one engagement we can't be late for. Old Mrs Hodgson is an absolute pet – she'd be terribly hurt if we let her supper spoil.'

I nodded. 'You're right, my girl, that mustn't happen. But I've got only three calls this afternoon and Tristan's doing the evening. I can't see anything going wrong.'

This nervousness about a simple action like going out for a meal might be incomprehensible to the layman but to vets and their wives it was very real, particularly in those days of one or two-man practices. The idea of somebody preparing a meal for me then waiting in vain for me to turn up was singularly horrifying but it happened to all of us occasionally.

It remained a gnawing worry whenever Helen and I were asked out; especially to somebody like the Hodgsons. Mr Hodgson was a particularly likeable old farmer, short-sighted to the point of semi-blindness, but the eyes which peered through the thick glasses were always friendly. His wife was just as kind and she had looked at me quizzically when I had visited the farm two days ago.

'Does it make you feel hungry, Mr Herriot?'

'It does indeed, Mrs Hodgson. It's a marvellous sight.'

I was washing my hands in the farm kitchen and stealing a glance at a nearby table where all the paraphernalia of the family pig-killing lay in their full glory. Golden rows of pork pies, spareribs, a mound of newly made sausages, jars of brawn. Great pots were being filled with lard, newly rendered in the fireside oven.

She looked at me thoughtfully. 'Why don't you bring Mrs Herriot round one night and help us eat it?'

'Well that's most kind of you and I'd love to, but . . .'

'Now then, no buts!' She laughed. 'You know there's far too much stuff here – we have to give so much away.'

This was quite true. In the days when every farmer and many

of the townsfolk of Darrowby kept pigs for home consumption, killing time was an occasion for feasting. The hams and sides were cured and hung up but the masses of offal and miscellaneous pieces had to be eaten at the time; and though farmers with big families could tackle it, others usually passed delicious parcels round their friends in the happy knowledge that there would be a reciprocation in due course.

'Well, thanks, Mrs Hodgson,' I said. 'Tuesday evening, then, seven o'clock.'

And here I was on Tuesday afternoon heading confidently into the country with the image of Mrs Hodgson's supper hanging before me like a vision of the promised land. I knew what it would be; a glorious mixed grill of spareribs, onions, liver and pork fillet garlanded with those divine farm sausages which are seen no more. It was something to dream about.

In fact I was still thinking about it when I drew into Edward Wiggin's farmyard. I walked over to the covered barn and looked in at my patients – a dozen half grown bullocks resting on the deep straw. I had to inject these fellows with Blackleg vaccine. If I didn't it was a fair bet that one or more of them would be found dead due to infection with the deadly Clostridium which dwelt in the pastures of that particular farm.

It was a common enough disease and stockholders had recognised it for generations and had resorted to some strange practices to prevent it; such as running a seton – a piece of twine or bandage – through the dewlap of the animal. But now we had an efficient vaccine.

I was thinking I'd be here for only a few minutes because Mr Wiggin's man, Wilf, was an expert beast catcher; then I saw the farmer coming across the yard and my spirits sank. He was carrying his lassoo. Wilf, by his side, rolled his eyes briefly heavenwards when he saw me. He too clearly feared the worst.

We went into the barn and Mr Wiggin began the painstaking process of arranging his long, white rope, while we watched him gloomily. He was a frail little man in his sixties and had spent some years of his youth in America. He didn't talk a lot about it but everybody in time gained the impression that he had been a sort of cowboy over there and indeed he talked in a soft Texan drawl and seemed obsessed with the mystique of the ranch and the open range. Anything to do with the Wild West was near to his heart and nearest of all was his lassoo.

You could insult Mr Wiggin with many things and he wouldn't turn a hair but question his ability to snare the wildest bovine with a single twirl of his rope and the mild little man could explode into anger. And the unfortunate thing was that he was no good at it.

Mr Wiggin had now got a long loop dangling from his hand and he began to whirl it round his head as he crept towards the nearest bullock. When he finally made his cast the result was as expected; the rope fell limply half way along the animal's back and dropped on to the straw.

'Tarnation!' said Mr Wiggin and started again. He was a man of deliberate movements and there was something maddening in the way he methodically assembled his rope again. It seemed an age before he once more advanced on a bullock with the rope whirring round his head.

'Bugger it!' Wilf grunted as the loop end lashed him across the face.

His boss turned on him. 'Keep out of the dadblasted road, Wilf,' he said querulously. 'I gotta start again now.'

This time he didn't even make contact with the animal and as he retrieved his lassoo from the straw Wilf and I leaned wearily against the wall of the barn.

Yet again the whizz of the rope and a particularly ambitious throw which sent it high into the criss-cross of beams in the roof where it stuck. The farmer tugged at it several times in vain.

'Goldurn it, it's got round a nail up there. Slip across the yard and fetch a ladder, Wilf.'

As I waited for the ladder then watched Wilf climbing into the shadowy heights of the barn I pondered on Mr Wiggin. The way he spoke, the expressions he used were familiar to most Yorkshire folk since they filtered continually across the Atlantic in films and books. In fact there were dark mutterings that Mr

Wiggin had learned them that way and had never been near a ranch in his life. There was no way of knowing.

At last the rope was retrieved, the ladder put away, and the little man went into action once more. He missed again but one of the bullocks got its foot in the loop and for a few moments the farmer hung on with fierce determination as the animal produced a series of piston-like kicks to rid itself of the distraction. And as I watched the man's lined face set grimly, the thin shoulders jerking, it came to me that Mr Wiggin wasn't just catching a beast for injection; he was roping a steer, the smell of the prairie was in his nostrils, the cry of the coyote in his ears.

It didn't take long for the bullock to free itself and with a grunt of 'Ornery crittur!' Mr Wiggin started again. And as he kept on throwing his rope ineffectually I was uncomfortably aware that time was passing and that our chances of doing our job were rapidly diminishing. When you have to handle a bunch of young beasts the main thing is not to upset them. If Mr Wiggin hadn't been there we would have penned them quietly in a corner and Wilf would have moved among them and caught their noses in his powerful fingers.

They were thoroughly upset. They had been peacefully chewing the cud or having a mouthful of hay from the rack but now, goaded by the teasing rope, were charging around like racehorses. Wilf and I watched in growing despair as Mr Wiggin for once managed to get a loop round one of them, but it was too wide and slipped down and round the body. The bullock shook it off with an angry bellow then went off at full gallop, bucking and kicking. I looked at the throng of frenzied creatures milling past; it was getting more like a rodeo every minute.

And it was a disastrous start to the afternoon. I had seen a couple of dogs at the surgery after lunch and it had been nearly two thirty when I set out. It was now nearly four o'clock and I hadn't done a thing.

And I don't think I ever would have if fate hadn't stepped in. By an amazing fluke Mr Wiggin cast his loop squarely over the horns of a shaggy projectile as it thundered past him, the rope tightened on the neck and Mr Wiggin on the other end flew gracefully through the air for about twenty feet till he crashed into a wooden feeding trough.

We rushed to him and helped him to his feet. Badly shaken but uninjured he looked at us.

'Doggone, I jest couldn't hold the blame thing,' he murmured. 'Reckon I'd better sit down in the house for a while. You'll have to catch that pesky lot yourselves.'

Back in the barn, Wilf whispered to me, 'By gaw it's an ill wind, guvnor. We can get on now. And maybe it'll make 'im forget that bloody lassoo for a bit.'

The bullocks were too excited to be caught by the nose but instead Wilf treated me to an exhibition of roping, Yorkshire style. Like many of the local stocksmen he was an expert with a halter and it fascinated me to see him dropping it on the head of a moving animal so that one loop fell behind the ears and the other snared the nose.

With a gush of relief I pulled the syringe and bottle of vaccine from my pocket and had the whole batch inoculated within twenty minutes.

Driving off I glanced at my watch and my pulse quickened as I saw it was a quarter to five. The afternoon had almost slipped away and there were still two more calls. But I had till seven o'clock and surely I wouldn't come across any more Mr Wiggins. And as the stone walls flipped past I ruminated again on that mysterious little man. Had he once been a genuine cowboy or was the whole thing fantasy?

I recalled that one Thursday evening Helen and I were leaving the Brawton cinema where we usually finished our half day; the picture had been a Western and just before leaving the dark interior I glanced along the back row and right at the far end I saw Mr Wiggin all on his own, huddled in the corner and looking strangely furtive.

Ever since then I have wondered. . . .

Five o'clock saw me hurrying into the smallholding belonging to the Misses Dunn. Their pig had cut its neck on a nail and my previous experience of this establishment suggested that it wouldn't be anything very serious.

These two maiden ladies farmed a few acres just outside Dollingsford village. They were objects of interest because they did most of the work themselves and in the process they lavished such affection on their livestock that they had become like domestic pets. The little byre held four cows and whenever I had to examine one of them I could feel the rough tongue of her neighbour licking at my back; their few sheep ran up to people in the fields and sniffed round their legs like dogs; calves sucked at your fingers, an ancient pony wandered around wearing a benign expression and nuzzling anyone within reach. The only exception among the amiable colony was the pig, Prudence, who was thoroughly spoiled.

I looked at her now as she nosed around the straw in her pen. She was a vast sow and the four-inch laceration in her neck muscles was obviously posing no threat to her life; but it was gaping and couldn't be left like that.

'I'll have to put a few stitches in there,' I said, and the big Miss Dunn gasped and put a hand to her mouth.

'Oh dear! Will it hurt her? I shan't be able to look, I'm afraid.'

She was a tall muscular lady in her fifties with a bright red face and often as I looked at her wide shoulders and the great arms with their bulging biceps I had the feeling that she could flatten me effortlessly with one blow if she so desired. But strangely she was nervous and squeamish about the realities of animal doctoring and it was always her little wisp of a sister who helped at lambings, calvings and the rest.

'Oh you needn't worry, Miss Dunn,' I replied. 'It'll be all over before she knows what's happening.' I climbed into the pen, went up to Prudence, and touched her gently on the neck.

Immediately the sow unleashed a petulant scream as though she had been stabbed with a hot iron and when I tried to give her back a friendly scratch the huge mouth opened again and the deafening sound blasted out. And this time she advanced on me threateningly. I stood my ground till the yawning cavern with its yellowed teeth was almost touching my leg then I put a hand on the rail and vaulted out of the pen.

'We'll have to get her into a smaller space,' I said. 'I'll never be able to stitch her in that big pen She has too much room to move around and she's too big to hold.'

Little Miss Dunn held up her hand. 'We have the very place. In the calf house across the yard. If we got her into one of those narrow stalls she wouldn't be able to turn round.'

'Fine!' I rubbed my hands. 'And I'll be able to do the stitching over the top from the passage. Let's get her over there.'

I opened the door and after a bit of poking and pushing Prudence ambled majestically out on to the cobbles of the yard. But there she stood, grunting sulkily, a stubborn glint in her little eyes, and when I leaned my weight against her back end it was like trying to move an elephant. She had no intention of moving any further; and that calf house was twenty yards away.

I stole a look at my watch. Five fifteen, and I didn't seem to be getting anywhere.

The little Miss Dunn broke into my thoughts. 'Mr Herriot, I know how we can get her across the yard.'

'You do?'

'Oh yes, Prudence has been naughty before and we have found a way of persuading her to move.'

I managed a smile. 'Great! How do you do it?'

'Well now,' and both sisters giggled, 'she is very fond of digestive biscuits '

'What's that?'

'She simply loves digestive biscuits.'

'She does?'

'Adores them!'

'Well, that's very nice,' I said 'But I don't quite see . . .'

The big Miss Dunn laughed. 'Just you wait and I'll show you.'

She began to stroll towards the house and it seemed to me that though those ladies were by no means typical Dales' farmers they did share the general attitude that time was of no consequence. The door closed behind her and I waited . . . and as the minutes ticked away I began to think she was brewing herself a cup of tea. In my mounting tension I turned away and gazed down over the hillside fields to where the grey roofs and old church tower of Dollingsford showed above the riverside trees. The quiet of the scene was in direct contrast to my mental state.

Just when I was giving up hope, big Miss Dunn reappeared carrying a long round paper container. She gave me a roguish smile as she held it up to me.

'These are what she likes. Now just watch.'

She produced a biscuit and threw it down on the cobbles a few feet in front of the sow. Prudence eyed it impassively for a few moments then without haste strolled forward, examined it carefully, and began to eat it.

When she had finished, big Miss Dunn glanced at me conspiratorially and threw another biscuit in front of her. The pig again moved on unhurriedly and started on the second course. This was gradually leading her towards the buildings across the yard but it was going to take a long time. I reckoned that each biscuit was advancing her about ten feet and the calf house would be all of twenty yards away, so allowing three minutes a biscuit it was going to take nearly twenty minutes to get there.

I broke out in a sweat at the thought, and my fears were justified because nobody was in the slightest hurry. Especially Prudence who slowly munched each titbit then snuffled around picking up every crumb while the ladies smiled down at her fondly.

'Look,' I stammered. 'Do you think you could throw the biscuits a bit further ahead of her ... just to save time, I mean?'

Little Miss Dunn laughed gaily. 'Oh we've tried that, but she's such a clever old darling. She knows she'll get less that way.'

To demonstrate she threw the next biscuit about fifteen feet away from the pig but the massive animal surveyed it with a cynical expression and didn't budge until it was kicked back to the required spot. Miss Dunn was right; Prudence wasn't so daft.

So I just had to wait, gritting my teeth as I watched the

agonising progress. I was almost at screaming point at the end though the others were thoroughly enjoying themselves. But at last the final biscuit was cast into the calf pen, the pig made her leisurely way inside and the ladies, with triumphant giggles, closed the door behind her.

I leapt forward with my needle and suture silk and of course as soon as I laid a finger on her skin Prudence set up an almost unbearable nonstop squeal of rage. Big Miss Dunn put her hands over her ears and fled in terror but her little sister stayed with me bravely and passed me my scissors and dusting powder whenever I asked in sign language above the din.

My head was still ringing as I drove away, but that didn't worry me as much as the time. It was six o'clock.

31

Tensely I assessed my position. The next and final visit was only a couple of miles away – I could make it in ten minutes. Then say twenty minutes on the farm, fifteen minutes back to Darrowby, a lightning wash and change and I could still be pushing my knees under Mrs Hodgson's table by seven o'clock.

And the next job wasn't a long one; just a bull to ring. Nowadays, since the advent of Artificial Insemination, there aren't many bulls about – only the big dairy men and pedigree breeders keep them – but in the thirties nearly every farmer had one, and inserting rings in their noses was a regular job. The rings were put in when they were about a year old and were necessary to restrain the big animals when they had to be led around.

I was immensely relieved when I arrived to find the gaunt figure of old Ted Buckle the farmer and his two men waiting for me in the yard. A classical way for a vet to waste time is to go hollering around the empty buildings then do more of the same out in the empty fields, waving madly, trying to catch the eye of a dot on the far horizon.

'Now then, young man,' Ted said, and even that short phrase took a fair time to come out. To me, the old man was a constant delight; speaking the real old Yorkshire – which you seldom hear now and which I won't try to reproduce here – with slow deliberation as though he were savouring every syllable as much as I was enjoying listening to him. 'You've come, then.'

'Yes, Mr Buckle, and I'm glad to see you're ready and waiting for me.'

'Aye, ah doan't like keepin' you fellers hangin' about.' He turned to his men. 'Now then, lads, go into that box and get haud'n that big lubber for Mr Herriot.'

The 'lads', Ernest and Herbert, who were both in their sixties, shuffled into the bull's loose box and closed the door after them. There were a few seconds of muffled banging against the wood, a couple of bellows and the occasional Anglo-Saxon expression from the men, then silence.

'Ah think they have 'im now,' Ted murmured and, not for the first time, I looked wonderingly at his wearing apparel. I had never seen him in anything else but that hat and coat in the time I had known him. With regard to the coat, which countless years ago must have been some kind of mackintosh, two things puzzled me: why he put it on and how he put it on. The long tatter of unrelated ribbons tied round the middle with binder twine could not possibly afford him any protection from the elements and how on earth did he know which were the sleeve holes among all the other apertures? And the hat, an almost crownless trilby from the early days of the century whose brim drooped vertically in sad folds over ears and eyebrows; it seemed incredible that he actually hung the thing up on a peg each night and donned it again in the morning.

Maybe the answer was to be found in the utterly serene humorous eyes which looked out from the skeleton-thin face. Nothing changed for Ted and the passage of a decade was a fleeting thing. I remember him showing me the old-fashioned 'reckon' which held the pans and kettles over the fire on his farm kitchen. He pointed out the row of holes where you could adjust it for large pans or small as though it were some modern invention.

'Aye, it's a wonderful thing, and t'lad that put it in for me made a grand job!'

'When was that, Mr Buckle?'

'It was eighteen ninety-seven. Ah remember it well. He was a right good workman was t'lad.'

But the men had reappeared with the young bull on a halter and they soon had him held in the accepted position for ringing.

There was a ritual about this job, a set pattern as unvarying as a classical ballet. Ernest and Herbert pulled the bull's head over the half door and held it there by pulling on a shank on either side of the halter. The portable crush had not yet been invented and this arrangement with the bull inside the box and the men outside was adopted for safety's sake. The next step was to make a hole through the tough tissue at the extremity of the nasal septum with the special punch which I had ready in its box.

But first there was a little refinement which I had introduced myself. Though it was the general custom to punch the hole without any preliminaries I always had the feeling that the bull might not like it very much; so I used to inject a couple of c.c.'s of local anaesthetic into the nose before I started. I poised my syringe now and Ernest, holding the left shank, huddled back apprehensively against the door.

'Tha's standin' middlin' to t'side, Ernest,' Ted drawled. 'Doesta think he's goin' to jump on top o' tha?'

'Naw, naw.' The man grinned sheepishly and took a shorter hold of the rope.

But he jumped back to his former position when I pushed the needle into the gristle just inside the nostril because the bull let loose a sudden deep-throated bellow of anger and reared up above the door. Ted had delayed ringing this animal; he was nearly eighteen months and very big.

'Haud 'im, lads,' Ted murmured as the two men clung to the

ropes. 'That's right – he'll settle down shortly.'

And he did. With his chin resting on the top of the door, held by the ropes on either side, he was ready for the next act. I pushed my punch into the nose, gripped the handles and squeezed. I never felt much like a professional gentleman when I did this, but at least my local had worked and the big animal didn't stir as the jaws of the instrument clicked together, puncturing a small round hole in the hard tissue.

The next stage in the solemn rite was unfolded as I unwrapped the bronze ring from its paper covering, took out the screw and opened the ring wide on its hinge. I waited for the inevitable words.

Ted supplied them. 'Take tha' cap off, Herbert. Tha woan't catch caud just for a minute.'

It was always a cap. A big bucket, a basin would have been more practical to hold that stupid, tiny screw and equally foolish little screwdriver, but it was always a cap. And a greasy old cap such as Herbert now removed from his polished pate.

My next step would be to slip the ring through the hole I had made, close it, insert the screw and tighten it up. That was where the cap came in; it was held under the ring to guard against sudden movements, because if the screw fell and was lost in the dirt and straw then all was lost. Then Ted would hand me the long rasp or file which every farmer had around somewhere and I would carefully smooth off the rim of the screw whether it needed it or not.

But this time there was to be a modification of the stereotyped little drama. As I stepped forward with my ring the young bull and I stood face to face and for a moment the wide set eyes under the stubby horns looked into mine. And as I reached out he must have moved slightly because the sharp end of the ring pricked him a little on the muzzle; the merest touch, but he seemed to take it as a personal insult because his mouth opened in an exasperated bawl and again he reared on his hind legs.

He was a well grown animal and in that position he looked very large indeed; and when his fore feet clumped down on the half door and the great rib cage loomed above us he was definitely formidable.

'The bugger's comin' over!' Ernest gasped and released his hold on the halter shank. He had never had much enthusiasm for the job and he abandoned it now without regret. Herbert was made of sterner stuff and he hung on grimly to his end as the bull thrashed above him, but after a cloven hoof had whizzed past his ear and another whistled just over his gleaming dome he too let go and fled.

Ted, untroubled as always, was well out of range and there remained only myself dancing in front of the door and gesticulating frantically at the bull in the vain hope that I might frighten him back whence he came; and the only thing that kept me there was the knowledge that every inch he scrambled out was taking me further from Mrs Hodgson's glorious supper.

I stood my ground until the snorting, bellowing creature was two thirds over, hanging grotesquely with the top of the door digging deep into his abdomen, then with a final plunge he was into the yard and I ran for cover. But the bull was not bent on mischief; he took one look at the open gate into the field and thundered through it like an express train.

From behind a stack of milk churns I watched sadly as he curveted joyously over the grass, revelling in his new found freedom. Bucking and kicking, tail in the air he headed for the far horizon where the wide pasture dipped to a beck which wandered along the floor of a shallow depression. And as he disappeared over the brow of the hill the last hope of my spareribs went with him.

'It'll tek us an hour to catch that bugger,' grunted Ernest gloomily.

I looked at my watch. Half past six. The bitter injustice of the whole thing overwhelmed me and I set up a wail of lamentation.

'Yes, dammit, and I've got an appointment in Darrowby at seven o'clock!' I stamped over the cobbles for a moment or two then swung round on old Ted. 'I'll never make it now . . . I'll have to ring my wife . . . have you got a phone?'

Ted's drawl was lazier than ever. 'Nay, we 'aven't got no phone. Ah don't believe in them things.' He fished out a tobacco

216

tin from his pocket, unscrewed the lid and produced a battered timepiece which he scrutinised without haste. 'Any road, there's nowt to stop ye bein' back i' Darrowby by seven.'

'But . . . but . . . that's impossible . . . and I can't keep these people waiting . . . I must get to a phone.'

'Doan't get s'flustered, young man.' The old man's long face creased into a soothing smile. 'Ah tell ye you won't be late.'

I waved my arms around. 'But he's just said it'll take an hour to catch that bull!'

'Fiddlesticks! Ernest allus talks like that . . . 'e's never 'appy unless 'e's miserable. Ah'll get bull in i' five minutes.'

'Five minutes! That's ridiculous! I'll . . . I'll drive down the road to the nearest phone box while you're catching him.'

'You'll do nowt of t'sort, lad.' Ted pointed to a stone water trough against the wall. 'Go and sit thissen down and think of summat else . . . ah'll only be five minutes.'

Wearily I sank on to the rough surface and buried my face in my hands. When I looked up the old man was coming out of the byre and in front of him ambled a venerable cow. By the number of rings on the long curving horns she must have been well into her teens; the gaunt pelvic bones stood out like a hatstand and underneath her a pendulous udder almost touched the ground.

'Get out there awd lass,' Ted said and the old cow trotted into the field, her udder swinging gently at each step. I watched her until she had disappeared over the hill, then turned to see Ted throwing cattle cake into a bucket.

He strolled through the gate and as I gazed uncomprehendingly he began to beat the bucket with a stick. At the same time he raised his voice in a reedy tenor and called out across the long stretch of green.

'Cush, cush!' he cried. 'Cush, pet, cush!'

Almost immediately the cow reappeared over the brow and just behind her the bull. I looked with wonder as Ted banged on his bucket and the cow broke into a stiff gallop with my patient close by her side. When she reached the old man she plunged her head in among the cake while the bull, though he was as big as she, pushed his nose underneath her and seized

217

one of her teats in his great mouth. It was an absurd sight but she didn't seem to mind as the big animal, almost on his knees, sucked away placidly.

In fact it was like a soothing potion because when the cow was led inside he followed; and he made no complaint as I slipped the ring in his nose and fastened it in with the screw which mercifully had survived inside Herbert's cap.

'Quarter to seven!' I panted happily as I jumped into the driving seat. 'I'll get there in time now.' I could see Helen and me standing on the Hodgson's step and the door opening and the heavenly scent of the spareribs and onions drifting out from the kitchen.

I looked again at the scarecrow figure with the hat brim drooping over the calm eyes. 'You did a wonderful job there, Mr Buckle. I wouldn't have believed it if I hadn't seen it. It was amazing how that bull followed the cow like that.'

The old man smiled and I had a sudden surging impression of the wisdom in that quiet mind.

'There's nowt amazin' about it, lad, it's most nat'ral thing in t'world. That's 'is mother.'

32

I slowed down and gazed along the farm lane. That was Tristan's car parked against the byre and inside, behind that green door, he was calving a cow. Because Tristan's student days were over. He was a fully fledged veterinary surgeon now and the great world of animal doctoring with all its realities stretched ahead.

Not for long, though, because like many others he was bound for the army and would leave soon after myself. But it wouldn't be so bad for Tristan because at least he would be doing his own job. When Siegfried and I had volunteered for service there had been no need for our profession in the army so we had gone into R.A.F. aircrew which was the only branch open to our 'reserved occupation'. But when it came to Tristan's turn the fighting had escalated in the far east and they were crying out for vets to doctor the horses, mules, cattle, camels.

The timing suggested that the Gods were looking after him as usual. In fact I think the Gods love people like Tristan who sway effortlessly before the winds of fate and spring back with a smile, looking on life always with blithe optimism. Anyway it seemed natural and inevitable that whereas Siegfried and I as second class aircraftmen pounded the parade ground for weary hours Captain Tristan Farnon sailed off to the war in style.

But in the meantime I was glad of his help. After my departure he would run things with the aid of an assistant, then, when he left, the practice would be in the hands of two strangers till we returned. It seemed strange but everything was impermanent at that time.

I drew up and looked thoughtfully at the car. This was Mark Dowson's place and when I had rung the surgery from out in the country Helen told me about this calving. I didn't want to butt in and fuss but I couldn't help wondering how Tristan was getting on, because Mr Dowson was a dour, taciturn character who wouldn't hesitate to come down on the young man if things went wrong.

Still, I hadn't anything to worry about because since he qualified Tristan was doing fine. The farmers had always liked him during his sporadic visits as a student but now that he was on the job regularly the good reports were coming in thick and fast.

'I'll tell tha, that young feller does work! Doesn't spare 'imself,' or 'Ah've never seen a lad put his 'eart and soul into his job like this 'un.' And one man drew me to one side and muttered, 'He meks some queer noises but he does try. I think he'd kill 'isself afore he'd give up.'

That last remark made me think. Tristan's forte was certainly not brute effort and I had been a bit bewildered at some of the

219

comments till I began to remember some of my experiences with him in his student days. He had always applied his acute intelligence to any situation in his own particular way and the way he reacted to the little accidents of country practice led me to believe he was operating a system.

The first time I saw this in action was when he was standing by the side of a cow watching me pulling milk from a teat. Without warning the animal swung round and brought an unyielding cloven hoof down on his foot. This is a common and fairly agonising experience and before the days of steel-tipped wellingtons I have frequently had the skin removed from my toes in neat parchment-like rolls. When it happened to me I was inclined to hop around and swear a bit and my performance was usually greeted with appreciative laughter from the farmers. Tristan, however, handled it differently.

He gasped, leaned with bowed head against the cow's pelvic bone for a moment then opened his mouth wide and emitted a long groan. Then, as the cowman and I stared at him, he reeled over the cobbles dragging the damaged limb uselessly behind him. Arrived at the far wall he collapsed against it, face on the stone, still moaning pitifully.

Thoroughly alarmed, I rushed to his aid. This must be a fracture and already my mind was busy with plans to get him to hospital with all possible speed. But he revived rapidly and when we left the byre ten minutes later he was tripping along with no trace of a limp. And I did notice one thing; nobody had laughed at him, he had received only sympathy and commiseration.

This sort of thing happened in other places. He sustained a few mild kicks, he was crushed between cows, he met with many of the discomforts which are part of our life and he reacted in the same histrionic way. And how it paid off! To a man, the farmers exhibited the deepest concern when he went into his act and there was something more; it actually improved his image. I was pleased about that because impressing Yorkshire farmers isn't the easiest task and if Tristan's method worked it was all right with me.

But I smiled to myself as I sat outside the farm. I couldn't see Mr Dowson being affected by any sign of suffering. I had had my knocks there in the past and he obviously hadn't cared a damn.

On an impulse I drove down the lane and walked into the byre. Tristan, stripped off and soaped, was just inserting an arm into a large red cow while the farmer, pipe in hand, was holding the tail. My colleague greeted me with a pleasant smile but Mr Dowson just nodded curtly.

'What have you got, Triss?' I asked.

'Both legs back,' he replied. 'And they're a long way in. Look at the length of her pelvis.'

I knew what he meant. It wasn't a difficult presentation but it could be uncomfortable in these long cows. I leaned back against the wall; I might as well see how he fared.

He braced himself and reached as far forward as he could, and just then the cow's flanks bulged as she strained hard against him. This is never very nice; the powerful contractions of the uterus squeeze the arm relentlessly between calf and pelvis and you have to grit your teeth till it passes off.

Tristan, however, went a little further.

'Ooh! Aah! Ouch!' he cried. Then as the animal still kept up the pressure he went into a gasping groan. When she finally relaxed he stood there quite motionless for a few seconds, his head hanging down as though the experience had drained him of all his strength.

The farmer drew on his pipe and regarded him impassively. Throughout the years I had known Mr Dowson I had never seen any particular emotion portrayed in those hard eyes and craggy features. In fact it had always seemed to me that I could have dropped down dead in front of him and he wouldn't even blink.

My colleague continued his struggle and the cow, entering into the spirit of the game, fought back with a will. Some animals will stand quietly and submit to all kinds of internal interference but this was a strainer; every movement of the arm within her was answered by a violent expulsive effort. I had been through it a hundred times and I could almost feel the grinding pressure on the wrist, the helpless numbing of the fingers.

Tristan showed what he thought about it all by a series of heart-rending sounds. His repertoire was truly astounding and he ranged from long harrowing moans through shrill squeals to an almost tearful whimpering.

At first Mr Dowson appeared oblivious to the whole business, puffing smoke, glancing occasionally through the byre door, scratching at the bristle on his chin. But as the minutes passed his eyes were dragged more and more to the suffering creature before him until his whole attention was riveted on the young man.

And in truth he was worth watching because Tristan added to his vocal performance an extraordinary display of facial contortions. He sucked in his cheeks, rolled his eyes, twisted his lips, did everything in fact but wiggle his ears. And there was no doubt he was getting through to Mr Dowson. As the noises and grimaces became more extravagant the farmer showed signs of growing uneasiness; he darted anxious glances at my colleague and occasionally his pipe trembled violently. Like me, he clearly thought some dreadful climax was at hand.

As if trying to bring matters to a head the cow started to build up a supreme effort. She straddled her legs wide, grunted deeply and went into a prolonged heave. As her back arched Tristan opened his mouth wide in a soundless protest then little panting cries began to escape him. This, I thought, was his most effective ploy yet; a long drawn 'Aah . . . aah . . . aah . . .' creeping gradually up the scale and building increasing tension in his audience. My toes were curling with apprehension when, with superb timing, he released a sudden piercing scream.

That was when Mr Dowson cracked. His pipe had almost wobbled from his mouth but now he stuffed it into his pocket and rushed to Tristan's side.

'Ista all right, young man?' he enquired hoarsely.

My colleague, his face a mask of anguish, did not reply.

The farmer tried again. 'Will ah get you a cup o' tea?'

For a moment Tristan made no response, then, eyes closed, he nodded dumbly.

Mr Dowson scampered eagerly from the byre and within minutes returned with a steaming mug. After that I had to shake my head to dispel the feeling of unreality. It couldn't be true, this vision of the hard-bitten farmer feeding the tea to the young man in sips, cradling the lolling head in a horny hand. Tristan was still inside the cow, still apparently semi-conscious with pain but submitting helplessly to the farmer's ministrations.

With a sudden lunge he produced one of the calf's legs and as he flopped against the cow's rump he was rewarded with another long gulp of tea. After the first leg the rest wasn't so bad and the second leg and the calf itself soon followed.

As the little creature landed wriggling on the floor, Tristan collapsed on his knees beside it and extended a trembling hand towards a pile of hay, prepared to give the new arrival a rub down.

Mr Dowson would have none of it.

'George!' he bellowed to one of his men in the yard. 'Get in 'ere and wisp this calf!' Then solicitously to Tristan, 'You maun come into t'house, lad, and have a drop o' brandy. You're about all in.'

The dream continued in the farm kitchen and I watched disbelievingly as my colleague fought his way back to health and strength with the aid of several stiff measures of Martell Three Star. I had never had treatment like this and a wave of envy swept over me as I wondered whether it was worth adopting Tristan's system.

But I still have never found the courage to try it.

33

It was strange, but somehow the labels on the calves' backs made them look even more pathetic; the auction mart labels stuck roughly with paste on the hairy rumps, stressing the little creatures' role as helpless merchandise.

As I lifted one sodden tail and inserted the thermometer a thin whitish diarrhoea trickled from the rectum and streamed down the thighs and hocks.

'It's the old story, I'm afraid, Mr Clark,' I said.

The farmer shrugged and dug his thumbs under his braces. In the blue overalls and peaked porter's cap he always wore he didn't look much like a farmer and for that matter this place did not greatly resemble a farm; the calves were in a converted railway wagon and all around lay a weird conglomeration of rusting agricultural implements, pieces of derelict cars, broken chairs. 'Aye, it's a beggar isn't it? I wish I didn't have to buy calves in markets but you can't always find 'em on t'farms when you want them. This lot looked all right when I got them two days since.'

'I'm sure they did.' I looked at the five calves, arch-backed, trembling, miserable. 'But they've had a tough time and it's showing now. Taken from their mothers at a week old, carted for miles in a draughty wagon, standing for most of the day at the mart then the final journey here on a cold afternoon. They didn't have a chance.'

'Well ah gave them a good bellyful of milk as soon as they came. They looked a bit starved and ah thought it would warm them up.'

'Yes, you'd think it would, Mr Clark, but really their stomachs weren't in a fit state to accept rich food like that when they were cold and tired. Next time if I were you I'd just give them a drink of warm water with maybe a little glucose and make them comfortable till next day.'

'White scour' they called it. It killed countless thousands of calves every year and the name always sent a chill through me because the mortality rate was depressingly high.

I gave each of them a shot of E coli antiserum. Most authorities said it did no good and I was inclined to agree with them. Then I rummaged in my car boot and produced a packet of our astringent powders of chalk, opium and catechu.

'Here, give them one of these three times a day, Mr Clark,' I said. I tried to sound cheerful but I'm sure my tone lacked conviction. Whiskered veterinary surgeons in top hats and tail coats had been prescribing chalk opium and catechu a hundred years ago and though it might have been helpful in mild diarrhoea it was almost useless against the lethal bacterial enteritis of white scour. It was a waste of time just trying to dry up the diarrhoea; what was wanted was a drug which would knock out the vicious bugs which caused it, but there wasn't such a thing around.

However there was one thing which we vets of those days used to do which is sometimes neglected since the arrival of the modern drugs; we attended to the comfort and nursing of the animals. The farmer and I wrapped each calf in a big sack which went right round its body and was fastened with binder twine round the ribs, in front of the brisket and under the tail. Then I fussed round the shed, plugging up draught holes, putting up a screen of straw bales between the calves and the door.

Before I left I took a last look at them; there was no doubt they were warm and she tered now. They would need every bit of help with only my astringent powders fighting for them.

I didn't see them again until the following afternoon. Mr Clark was nowhere around so I went over to the railway wagon and opened the half door.

This, to me, is the thing that lies at the very heart of veterinary practice; the wondering and worrying about how your patient is progressing then the long moment when you open that door and find out. I rested my elbows on the timbers and looked inside. The calves were lying quite motionless on their sides, in fact I had to look closely to make sure they were not dead. I banged the door behind me with deliberate force but not a head was raised.

Walking through the deep straw and looking down at the outstretched animals, each in his rough sacking jacket, I swore to myself. It looked as though the whole lot was going to perish. Great, great, I thought as I kicked among the straw – not just one or two but a hundred per cent death rate this time.

'Well you don't look very 'opeful, young man.' Mr Clark's head and shoulders loomed over the half door.

I dug my hands into my pockets. 'No, damn it, I'm not. They've gone down really fast, haven't they?'

'Aye, it's ower wi' them all right. I've just been in t'house ringing Mallock.'

The knacker man's name was like the pealing of a mournful bell. 'But they're not dead yet,' I said.

'No, but it won't be long. Mallock allus gives a bob or two more if he can get a beast alive. Makes fresher dog meat, he says.'

I didn't say anything and I must have looked despondent because the farmer gave a wry smile and came over to me.

'It isn't your fault, lad. I know all about this dang white scour. If you get the right bad sort there's nothing anybody can do. And you can't blame me for tryin' to get a bit back – I've got to make the best of a bad job.'

'Oh I know,' I said. 'I'm just disappointed I can't have a go at them with this new medicine.'

'What's that, then?'

I took the tin from my pocket and read the label. 'It's called M and B 693, or sulphapyridine, to give it its scientific name. Just came in the post this morning. It's one of a completely new range of drugs – they're called the sulphonamides and we've never had anything like them before. They're supposed to actually kill certain germs, such as the organisms which cause scour.'

Mr Clark took the tin from me and removed the lid. 'A lot of little blue tablets, eh? Well ah've seen a few wonder cures for this ailment but none of 'em's much good – this'll be another, I'll bet.'

'Could be,' I said. 'But there's been a lot of discussion about these sulphonamides in our veterinary journals. They're not quack remedies, they're a completely fresh field. I wish I could have tried them on your calves.'

'Well look at them.' The farmer gazed gloomily over the five still bodies. 'Their eyes are goin' back in their heads. Have you ever seen calves like that get better?'

'No, I haven't, but I'd still like to have a go.'

As I spoke a tall-sided wagon rumbled into the yard. A sprightly, stocky man descended from the driver's seat and came over to us.

'By gaw, Jeff,' said Mr Clark. 'You 'aven't been long.'

'Naw, they got me on t'phone at Jenkinson's, just down t' road.' He gave me a smile of peculiar sweetness.

I studied Jeff Mallock as I always did with a kind of wonder. He had spent the greater part of his forty odd years delving in decomposing carcases, slashing nonchalantly with his knife at tuberculous abscesses, wallowing in infected blood and filthy uterine exudates yet he remained a model of health and fitness. He had the clear eyes and the smooth pink skin of a twenty-year-old and the effect was heightened by the untroubled serenity of his expression. To the best of my knowledge Jeff never took any hygienic precautions such as washing his hands and I have seen him enjoying a snack on his premises, seated on a heap of bones and gripping a cheese and onion sandwich with greasy fingers.

He peered over the door at the calves. 'Yes, yes, a clear case of stagnation of t'lungs. There's a lot of it about right now.'

Mr Clark looked at me narrowly. 'Lungs? You never said owt about lungs, young man.' Like all farmers he had complete faith in Jeff's instant diagnosis.

I mumbled something. I had found it useless to argue this point. The knacker man's amazing ability to tell at a glance the cause of an animal's illness or death was a frequent source of embarrassment to me. No examination was necessary – he just knew, and of all his weird catalogue of diseases stagnation of t'lungs was the favourite.

He turned to the farmer. 'Well, ah'd better shift 'em now, Willie. Reckon they won't last much longer.'

227

I bent down and lifted the head of the nearest calf. They were all shorthorns, three roans, a red and this one which was pure white. I passed my fingers over the hard little skull, feeling the tiny horn buds under the rough hair. When I withdrew my hand the head dropped limply on to the straw and it seemed to me that there was something of finality and resignation in the movement.

My thoughts were interrupted by the roar of Jeff's engine. He was backing his wagon round to the door of the calf house and as the high unpainted boards darkened the entrance the atmosphere of gloom deepened. These little animals had suffered two traumatic journeys in their short lives. This was to be the last, the most fateful and the most sordid.

When the knacker man came in he stood by the farmer, looking at me as I squatted in the straw among the prostrate creatures. They were both waiting for me to quit the place, leaving my failure behind me.

'You know, Mr Clark,' I said, 'even if we could save one of them it would help to reduce your loss.'

The farmer regarded me expressionlessly. 'But they're all dyin', lad. You said so yourself.'

'Yes, I did, I know, but the circumstances could be a bit different today.'

'Ah know what it is.' He laughed suddenly. 'You've got your heart set on havin' a go with them little tablets, haven't you?'

I didn't answer but looked up at him with a mute appeal.

He was silent for a few moments then he put a hand on Mallock's shoulder. 'Jeff, if this young feller is that concerned about ma stock I'll 'ave to humour 'im. You're not bothered, are you?'

'Nay, Willie, nay,' replied Jeff, completely unruffled, 'I can pick 'em up tomorrow, just as easy.'

'Right,' I said. 'Let's have a look at the instructions.' I fished out the pamphlet from the tin and read rapidly, working out the dose for the weight of the calves. 'We'll have to give them a loading dose first. I think twelve tablets per calf then six every eight hours after that.'

'How do you get 'em down their necks?' the farmer asked.

'We'll have to crush them and shake them up in water. Can we go into the house to do that?'

In the farm kitchen we borrowed Mrs Clark's potato masher and pounded the tablets until we had five initial doses measured out. Then we returned to the shed and began to administer them to the calves. We had to go carefully as the little creatures were so weak they had difficulty in swallowing, but the farmer held each head while I trickled the medicine into the side of the mouth.

Jeff enjoyed every minute of it. He showed no desire to leave but produced a pipe richly decorated with nameless tissues, leaned on the top of the half door and, puffing happily, watched us with tranquil eyes. He was quite unperturbed by his wasted journey and when we had finished he climbed into his wagon and waved to us cordially.

'I'll be back to pick 'em up in t'mornin', Willie,' he cried, quite without malice I'm sure. 'There's no cure for stagnation of t'lungs.'

I thought of his words next day as I drove back to the farm. He was just stating the fact; his supply of dog meat was merely being postponed for another twenty-four hours. But at least, I told myself, I had the satisfaction of having tried, and since I expected nothing I wasn't going to be disappointed.

As I pulled up in the yard Mr Clark walked over and spoke through the window. 'There's no need for you to get out of the car.' His face was a grim mask.

'Oh,' I said, the sudden lurch in my stomach belying my calm facade. 'Like that, is it?'

'Aye, come and look 'ere.' He turned and I followed him over to the shed. By the time the door creaked open a slow misery had begun to seep into me.

Unwillingly I gazed into the interior.

Four of the calves were standing in a row looking up at us with interest. Four shaggy, rough-jacketed figures, bright-eyed and alert. The fifth was resting on the straw, chewing absently at one of the strings which held his sack.

The farmer's weathered face split into a delighted grin. 'Well ah told you there was no need to get out of your car, didn't I? They don't need no vitnery, they're back to normal.'

I didn't say anything. This was something which my mind, as yet, could not comprehend. As I stared unbelievingly the fifth calf rose from the straw and stretched luxuriously.

'He's wraxin', d'you see?' cried Mr Clark. 'There's nowt much wrong wi' them when they do that.'

We went inside and I began to examine the little animals. Temperatures were normal, the diarrhoea had dried up, it was uncanny. As if in celebration the white calf which had been all but dead yesterday began to caper about the shed, kicking up his legs like a mustang.

'Look at that little bugger!' burst out the farmer. 'By gaw I wish I was as fit meself!'

I put the thermometer back in its tube and dropped it into my side pocket. 'Well, Mr Clark,' I said slowly, 'I've never seen anything like this. I still feel stunned.'

'Beats hen-racin', doesn't it,' the farmer said, wide-eyed, then he turned towards the gate as a wagon appeared from the lane. It was the familiar doom-burdened vehicle of Jeff Mallock.

The knacker man showed no emotion as he looked into the shed. In fact it was difficult to imagine anything disturbing those pink cheeks and placid eyes, but I fancied the puffs of blue smoke from his pipe came a little faster as he took in the scene. The pipe itself showed some fresh deposits on its bowl – some fragments of liver, I fancied, since yesterday.

When he had looked his fill he turned and strolled towards his wagon. On the way he gazed expansively around him and then at the dark clouds piling in the western sky.

'Ah think it'll turn to rain afore t'day's out, Willie,' he murmured.

I didn't know it at the time but I had witnessed the beginning of the revolution. It was my first glimpse of the tremendous therapeutic breakthrough which was to sweep the old remedies into oblivion. The long rows of ornate glass bottles with their carved stoppers and Latin inscriptions would not stand on the dispensary shelves much longer and their names, dearly familiar for many generations – Sweet Spirits of Nitre, Sal ammoniac, Tincture of Camphor – would be lost and vanish for ever.

This was the beginning and just around the corner a new wonder was waiting – Penicillin and the other antibiotics. At last we had something to work with, at last we could use drugs which we knew were going to do something.

All over the country, probably all over the world at that time, vets were having these first spectacular results, going through the same experience as myself; some with cows, some with dogs and cats, others with valuable racehorses, sheep, pigs in all kinds of environments. But for me it happened in that old converted railway wagon among the jumble of rusting junk on Willie Clark's farm.

Of course it didn't last – not the miraculous part of it anyway. What I had seen at Willie Clark's was the impact of something new on an entirely unsophisticated bacterial population, but it didn't go on like that. In time the organisms developed a certain amount of resistance and new and stronger sulphonamides and antibiotics had to be produced. And so the battle has continued. We have good results now but no miracles, and I feel I was lucky to be one of the generation which was in at the beginning when the wonderful things did happen.

Those five calves never looked behind them and the memory of them gives me a warm glow even now. Willie, of course, was overjoyed and even Jeff Mallock gave the occasion his particular accolade. As he drove away he called back to us:

'Them little blue tablets must have good stuff in 'em. They're fust things I've ever seen could cure stagnation of t'lungs.'

34

There was one marvellous thing about the set-up in Darrowby. I had the inestimable advantage of being a large animal practitioner with a passion for dogs and cats. So that although I spent most of my time in the wide outdoors of Yorkshire there was always the captivating background of the household pets to make a contrast.

I treated some of them every day and it made an extra interest in my life; interest of a different kind, based on sentiment instead of commerce and because of the way things were it was something I could linger over and enjoy. I suppose with a very intensive small animal practice it would be easy to regard the thing as a huge sausage machine, an endless procession of hairy forms to prod with hypodermic needles. But in Darrowby we got to know them all as individual entities.

Driving through the town I was able to identify my ex-patients without difficulty; Rover Johnson, recovered from his ear canker, coming out of the ironmongers with his mistress; Patch Walker, whose broken leg had healed beautifully, balanced happily on the back of his owner's coal wagon, or Spot Briggs who was a bit of a rake anyway and would soon be tearing himself again on barbed wire, ambling all alone across the market place cobbles in search of adventure. I got quite a kick out of recalling their ailments and mulling over their characteristics. Because they all had their own personalities and they were manifested in different ways.

One of these was their personal reaction to me and my treatment. Most dogs and cats appeared to bear me not the slightest ill will despite the fact that I usually had to do something disagreeable to them.

But there were exceptions and one of these was Magnus, the Miniature Dachshund from the Drovers' Arms.

He was in my mind now as I leaned across the bar counter.

'A pint of Smiths, please, Danny,' I whispered.

The barman grinned. 'Coming up, Mr Herriot.' He pulled at the lever and the beer hissed gently into the glass and as he passed it over the froth stood high and firm on the surface.

'That ale looks really fit tonight,' I breathed almost inaudibly.

'Fit? It's beautiful!' Danny looked fondly at the brimming glass. 'In fact it's a shame to sell it.'

I laughed, but pianissimo. 'Well it's nice of you to spare me a drop.' I took a deep pull and turned to old Mr Fairburn who was as always sitting at the far corner of the bar with his own fancy flower-painted glass in his hand.

'It's been a grand day, Mr Fairburn,' I murmured *sotto voce*. The old man put his hand to his ear. 'What's that you say?'

'Nice warm day it's been.' My voice was like a soft breeze sighing over the marshes.

I felt a violent dig at my back. 'What the heck's the matter with you, Jim? Have you got laryngitis?'

I turned and saw the tall bald-headed figure of Dr Allinson, my medical adviser and friend. 'Hello, Harry,' I cried. 'Nice to see you.' Then I put my hand to my mouth.

But it was too late. A furious yapping issued from the manager's office. It was loud and penetrating and it went on and on.

'Damn, I forgot,' I said wearily. 'There goes Magnus again.'

'Magnus? What are you talking about?'

'Well, it's a long story.' I took another sip at my beer as the din continued from the office. It really shattered the peace of the comfortable bar and I could see the regulars fidgeting and looking out into the hallway.

Would that little dog ever forget? It seemed a long time now since Mr Beckwith, the new young manager at the Drovers, had brought Magnus in to the surgery. He had looked a little apprehensive.

'You'll have to watch him, Mr Herriot.'

'What do you mean?'

'Well, be careful. He's very vicious.'

I looked at the sleek little form, a mere brown dot on the table. He would probably turn the scale at around six pounds. And I couldn't help laughing.

'Vicious? He's not big enough, surely.'

'Don't you worry!' Mr Beckwith raised a warning finger. 'I took him to the vet in Bradford where I used to manage the White Swan and he sank his teeth into the poor chap's finger.'

'He did?'

'He certainly did! Right down to the bone! By God I've never heard such language but I couldn't blame the man. There was blood all over the place. I had to help him to put a bandage on.'

'Mm, I see.' It was nice to be told before you had been bitten and not after. 'And what was he trying to do to the dog? Must have been something pretty major.'

'It wasn't you know. All I wanted was his nails clipping.'

'Is that all? And why have you brought him today?'

'Same thing.'

'Well honestly, Mr Beckwith,' I said, 'I think we can manage to cut his nails without bloodshed. If he'd been a Bull Mastiff or an Alsatian we might have had a problem, but I think that you and I between us can control a Miniature Dachshund.'

The manager shook his head. 'Don't bring me into it. I'm sorry, but I'd rather not hold him, if you don't mind.'

'Why not?'

'Well, he'd never forgive me. He's a funny little dog.'

I rubbed my chin. 'But if he's as difficult as you say and you can't hold him, what do you expect me to do?'

'I don't know, really . . . maybe you could sort of dope him . . . knock him out?'

'You mean a general anaesthetic? To cut his claws . . . ?'

'It'll be the only way, I'm afraid.' Mr Beckwith stared gloomily at the tiny animal. 'You don't know him.'

It was difficult to believe but it seemed pretty obvious that this canine morsel was the boss in the Beckwith home. In my experience many dogs had occupied this position but none as small as this one. Anyway, I had no more time to waste on this nonsense.

'Look,' I said. 'I'll put a tape muzzle on his nose and I'll have this job done in a couple of minutes.' I reached behind me for the nail clippers and laid them on the table, then I unrolled a length of bandage and tied it in a loop.

'Good boy, Magnus,' I said ingratiatingly as I advanced towards him.

The little dog eyed the bandage unwinkingly until it was almost touching his nose then, with a surprising outburst of ferocity, he made a snarling leap at my hand. I felt the draught on my fingers as a row of sparkling teeth snapped shut half an inch away, but as he turned to have another go my free hand clamped on the scruff of his neck.

'Right, Mr Beckwith,' I said calmly, 'I have him now. Just pass me that bandage again and I won't be long.'

But the young man had had enough. 'Not me!' he gasped. 'I'm off!' He turned the door handle and I heard his feet scurrying along the passage.

Ah well, I thought, it was probably best. With boss dogs my primary move was usually to get the owner out of the way. It was surprising how quickly these tough guys calmed down when they found themselves alone with a no-nonsense stranger who knew how to handle them. I could recite a list who were raving tearaways in their own homes but apologetic tail-waggers once they crossed the surgery threshold. And they were all bigger than Magnus.

Retaining my firm grip on his neck I unwound another foot of bandage and as he fought furiously, mouth gaping, lips retracted like a scaled-down Siberian wolf, I slipped the loop over his nose, tightened it and tied the knot behind his ears. His mouth was now clamped shut and just to make sure, I applied a second bandage so that he was well and truly trussed.

This was when they usually packed in and I looked confidently at the dog for signs of submission. But above the encircling white coils the eyes glared furiously and from within the little frame an enraged growling issued, rising and falling like the distant droning of a thousand bees.

Sometimes a stern word or two had the effect of showing them who was boss.

'Magnus!' I barked at him. 'That's enough! Behave yourself!' I gave his neck a shake to make it clear that I wasn't kidding but the only response was a sidelong squint of pure defiance from the slightly bulging eyes.

I lifted the clippers. 'All right,' I said wearily, 'if you won't have it one way you'll have it the other.' And I tucked him under one arm, seized a paw and began to clip.

He couldn't do a thing about it. He fought and wriggled but I had him as in a vice. And as I methodically trimmed the overgrown nails, wrathful bubbles escaped on either side of the bandage along with his splutterings. If dogs could swear I was getting the biggest cursing in history.

I did my job with particular care, taking pains to keep well away from the sensitive core of the claw so that he felt nothing, but it made no difference. The indignity of being mastered for once in his life was insupportable.

Towards the conclusion of the operation I began to change my tone. I had found in the past that once dominance has been established it is quite easy to work up a friendly relationship, so I started to introduce a wheedling note.

'Good little chap,' I cooed. 'That wasn't so bad, was it ?'

I laid down the clippers and stroked his head as a few more resentful bubbles forced their way round the bandage. 'All right, Magnus, we'll take your muzzle off now.' I began to loosen the knot. 'You'll feel a lot better then, won't you ?'

So often it happened that when I finally removed the restraint the dog would apparently decide to let bygones be bygones and in some cases would even lick my hand. But not so with Magnus. As the last turn of bandage fell from his nose he made another very creditable attempt to bite me.

'All right, Mr Beckwith,' I called along the passage, 'you can come and get him now.'

My final memory of the visit was of the little dog turning at the top of the surgery steps and giving me a last dirty look before his master led him down the street.

It said very clearly, 'Right, mate, I won't forget you.'

*   *   *

That had been weeks ago but ever since that day the very sound of my voice was enough to set Magnus yapping his disapproval. At first the regulars treated it as a big joke but now they had started to look at me strangely. Maybe they thought I had been cruel to the animal or something. It was all very embarrassing because I didn't want to abandon the Drovers; the bar was always cosy even on the coldest night and the beer very consistent.

Anyway if I had gone to another pub I would probably have started to do my talking in whispers and people would have looked at me even more strangely then.

How different it was with Mrs Hammond's Irish Setter. This started with an urgent phone call one night when I was in the bath. Helen knocked on the bathroom door and I dried off quickly and threw on my dressing gown. I ran upstairs and as soon as I lifted the receiver an anxious voice burst in my ear.

'Mr Herriot, it's Rock! He's been missing for two days and a man has just brought him back now. He found him in a wood with his foot in a gin trap. He must . . .' I heard a half sob at the end of the line. 'He must have been caught there all this time.'

'Oh, I'm sorry! Is it very bad?'

'Yes it is.' Mrs Hammond was the wife of one of the local bank managers and a capable, sensible woman. There was a pause and I imagined her determinedly gaining control of herself. When she spoke her voice was calm.

'Yes, I'm afraid it looks as though he'll have to have his foot amputated.'

'Oh, I'm terribly sorry to hear that.' But I wasn't really surprised. A limb compressed in one of those barbarous instruments for forty-eight hours would be in a critical state. These traps are now mercifully illegal but in those days they often provided me with the kind of jobs I didn't want and the kind of decisions I hated to make. Did you take a limb from an uncomprehending animal to keep it alive or did you bring down the merciful but final curtain of euthanasia? I was responsible for the fact that there were several three-legged dogs and cats running around Darrowby and though they seemed happy enough and their owners still had the pleasure of their pets, the thing, for me, was clouded with sorrow.

Anyway, I would do what had to be done.

'Bring him straight round, Mrs Hammond,' I said.

Rock was a big dog but he was the lean type of Setter and seemed very light as I lifted him on to the surgery table. As my arms encircled the unresisting body I could feel the rib cage sharply ridged under the skin.

'He's lost a lot of weight,' I said.

His mistress nodded. 'It's a long time to go without food. He ate ravenously when he came in, despite his pain.'

I put a hand beneath the dog's elbow and gently lifted the leg. The vicious teeth of the trap had been clamped on the radius and ulna but what worried me was the grossly swollen state of the foot. It was at least twice its normal size.

'What do you think, Mr Herriot?' Mrs Hammond's hands twisted anxiously at the handbag which every woman seemed to bring to the surgery irrespective of the circumstances.

I stroked the dog's head. Under the light, the rich sheen of the coat glowed red and gold. 'This terrific swelling of the foot. It's partly due to inflammation but also to the fact that the circulation was pretty well cut off for the time he was in the trap. The danger is gangrene – that's when the tissue dies and decomposes.'

'I know,' she replied. 'I did a bit of nursing before I married.'

Carefully I lifted the enormous foot. Rock gazed calmly in front of him as I felt around the metacarpals and phalanges, working my way up to the dreadful wound.

'Well, it's a mess,' I said, 'but there are two good things. First, the leg isn't broken. The trap has gone right down to the bone but there is no fracture. And second and more important, the foot is still warm.'

'That's a good sign?'

'Oh yes. It means there's still some circulation. If the foot had been cold and clammy the thing would have been hopeless. I would have had to amputate.'

'You think you can save his foot, then?'

I held up my hand. 'I don't know, Mrs Hammond. As I say, he still has some circulation but the question is how much. Some of this tissue is bound to slough off and things could look very nasty in a few days. But I'd like to try.'

I flushed out the wound with a mild antiseptic in warm water and gingerly explored the grisly depths. As I snipped away the pieces of damaged muscle and cut off the shreds and flaps of dead skin the thought was uppermost that it must be extremely unpleasant for the dog; but Rock held his head high and scarcely flinched. Once or twice he turned his head towards me enquiringly as I probed deeply and at times I felt his moist nose softly brushing my face as I bent over the foot, but that was all.

The injury seemed a desecration. There are few more beautiful dogs than an Irish Setter and Rock was a picture; sleek coated and graceful with silky feathers on legs and tail and a noble, gentle-eyed head. As the thought of how he would look without a foot drove into my mind I shook my head and turned quickly to lift the sulphanilamide powder from the trolley behind me. Thank heavens this was now available, one of the new revolutionary drugs, and I packed it deep into the wound with the confidence that it would really do something to keep down the infection. I applied a layer of gauze then a light bandage with a feeling of fatalism. There was nothing else I could do.

Rock was brought in to me every day. And every day he endured the same procedure; the removal of the dressing which was usually adhering to the wound to some degree, then the inevitable trimming of the dying tissues and the rebandaging. Yet, incredibly, he never showed any reluctance to come. Most of my patients came in very slowly and left at top speed, dragging their owners on the end of the leads; in fact some turned tail at the door, slipping their collar and sped down Trengate with their owners in hot pursuit. Dogs aren't so daft and there is doubtless a dentist's chair type of association about a vet's surgery.

Rock, however, always marched in happily with a gentle waving of his tail. In fact when I went into the waiting room and saw him sitting there he usually offered me his paw. This had always been a characteristic gesture of his but there seemed something uncanny about it when I bent over him and saw the white-swathed limb outstretched towards me.

After a week the outlook was grim. All the time the dead tissue had been sloughing and one night when I removed the dressing Mrs Hammond gasped and turned away. With her nursing training she had been very helpful, holding the foot this way and that intuitively as I worked, but tonight she didn't want to look.

I couldn't blame her. In places the white bones of the metacarpals could be seen like the fingers of a human hand with only random strands of skin covering them.

'Is it hopeless, do you think?' she whispered, still looking away.

I didn't answer for a moment as I felt my way underneath the foot. 'It does look awful, but do you know, I think we have reached the end of the road and are going to turn the corner soon.'

'How do you mean?'

'Well, all the under surface is sound and warm. His pads are perfectly intact. And do you notice, there's no smell tonight? That's because there is no more dead stuff to cut away. I really think this foot is going to start granulating.'

She stole a look. 'And do you think those . . . bones . . . will be covered over?'

'Yes, I do.' I dusted on the faithful sulphanilamide. 'It won't be exactly the same foot as before but it will do.'

And it turned out just that way. It took a long time but the new healthy tissue worked its way upwards as though determined to prove me right and when, many months later, Rock came into the surgery with a mild attack of conjunctivitis he proffered a courteous paw as was his wont. I accepted the civility and as we shook hands I looked at the upper surface of the foot. It was hairless, smooth and shining, but it was completely healed.

'You'd hardly notice it, would you?' Mrs Hammond said.

'That's right, it's marvellous. Just this little bare patch. And he walked in without a limp.'

Mrs Hammond laughed. 'Oh, he's quite sound on that leg now. And do you know, I really think he's grateful to you – look at him.'

I suppose the animal psychologists would say it was ridiculous even to think that the big dog realised I had done him a bit of good; that lolling-tongued open mouth, warm eyes and outstretched paw didn't mean anything like that.

Maybe they are right, but what I do know and cherish is the certainty that after all the discomforts I had put him through Rock didn't hold a thing against me.

I have to turn to the other side of the coin to discuss Timmy Butterworth. He was a wire-haired Fox Terrier who resided in Gimber's yard, one of the little cobbled alleys off Trengate, and the only time I had to treat him was one lunch time.

I had just got out of the car and was climbing the surgery steps when I saw a little girl running along the street, waving frantically as she approached. I waited for her and when she panted up to me her eyes were wide with fright.

'Ah'm Wendy Butterworth,' she gasped. 'Me mam sent me. Will you come to our dog?'

'What's wrong with him?'

'Me mam says he's et summat!'

'Poison?'

'Ah think so.'

It was less than a hundred yards away, not worth taking the car. I broke into a trot with Wendy by my side and within seconds we were turning into the narrow archway of the 'yard'. Our feet clattered along the tunnel-like passage then we emerged into one of the unlikely scenes which had surprised me so much when I first came to Darrowby; the miniature street with its tiny crowded houses, strips of garden, bow windows looking into each other across a few feet of cobbles. But I had no time to gaze around me today because Mrs Butterworth, stout, red-faced and very flustered was waiting for me.

'He's in 'ere, Mr Herriot!' she cried and threw wide the door of one of the cottages. It opened straight into the living room and I saw my patient sitting on the hearth rug looking somewhat thoughtful.

'What's happened, then?' I asked.

The lady clasped and unclasped her hands. 'I saw a big rat run down across t'yard yesterday and I got some poison to put down for 'im.' She gulped agitatedly. 'I mixed it in a saucer full o' porridge then somebody came to t'door and when ah came back, Timmy was just finishin' it off!'

The terrier's thoughtful expression had deepened and he ran his tongue slowly round his lips with the obvious reflection that that was the strangest porridge he had ever tasted.

I turned to Mrs Butterworth. 'Have you got the poison tin there?'

'Yes, here it is.' With a violently trembling hand she passed it to me.

I read the label. It was a well known name and the very look of it sounded a knell in my mind recalling the many dead and dying animals with which it was associated. Its active ingredient was zinc phosphide and even today with our modern drugs we are usually helpless once a dog has absorbed it.

I thumped the tin down on the table. 'We've got to make him vomit immediately! I don't want to waste time going back to the surgery – have you got any washing soda? If I push a few crystals down it'll do the trick.'

'Oh dear!' Mrs Butterworth bit her lip. 'We 'aven't such a thing in the house . . . is there anything else we could . . .'

'Wait a minute!' I looked across the table, past the piece of cold mutton, the tureen of potatoes and a jar of pickles. 'Is there any mustard in that pot?'

'Aye, it's full.'

Quickly I grabbed the pot, ran to the tap and diluted the mustard to the consistency of milk.

'Come on!' I shouted. 'Let's have him outside.'

I seized the astonished Timmy, whisked him from the rug, shot through the door and dumped him on the cobbles. Holding his body clamped tightly between my knees and his jaws close together with my left hand I poured the liquid mustard into the side of his mouth whence it trickled down to the back of his throat. There was nothing he could do about it, he had swallowed the disgusting stuff, and when about a tablespoon had gone down I released him.

After a single affronted glare at me the terrier began to retch then to lurch across the smooth stones. Within seconds he had deposited his stolen meal in a quiet corner.

'Do you think that's the lot?' I asked.

'That's it,' Mrs Butterworth replied firmly. 'I'll fetch a brush and shovel.'

Timmy, his short tail tucked down, slunk back into the house and I watched him as he took up his favourite position on the hearthrug. He coughed, snorted, pawed at his mouth, but he just couldn't rid himself of that dreadful taste; and increasingly it was obvious that he had me firmly tagged as the cause of all the trouble. As I left he flashed me a glance which said quite plainly, 'You rotten swine!'

There was something in that look which reminded me of Magnus from the Drovers, but the first sign that Timmy, unlike Magnus, wasn't going to be satisfied with vocal disapproval came within a few days. I was strolling meditatively down Trengate when a white missile issued from Gimber's Yard, nipped me on the ankle and disappeared as silently as he had come. I caught only a glimpse of the little form speeding on its short legs down the passage.

I laughed. Fancy his remembering! But it happened again and again and I realised that the little dog was indeed lying in wait for me. He never actually sank his teeth into me – it was a gesture more than anything – but it seemed to satisfy him to see me jump as he snatched briefly at my calf or trouser leg. I was a sitting bird because I was usually deep in thought as I walked down the street.

And when I thought about it, I couldn't blame Timmy. Looking at it from his point of view he had been sitting by his fireside digesting an unusual meal and minding his own business when a total stranger had pounced on him, hustled him from the comfort of his rug and poured mustard into him. It was outrageous and he just wasn't prepared to let the matter rest there.

For my part there was a certain satisfaction in being the object of a vendetta waged by an animal who would have been dead without my services. And unpleasantly dead because the victims of phosphorus poisoning had to endure long days and sometimes weeks of jaundice, misery and creeping debility before the inevitable end.

So I suffered the attacks with good grace. But when I remembered I crossed to the other side of the street to avoid the hazard of Gimber's Yard; and from there I could often see the little white dog peeping round the corner waiting for the moment when he would make me pay for that indignity.

Timmy, I knew, was one who would never forget.

35

I suppose there was a wry humour in the fact that my call-up papers arrived on my birthday, but I didn't see the joke at the time.

The event is preserved in my memory in a picture which is as clear to me today as when I walked into our 'dining room' that morning. Helen perched away up on her high stool at the end of the table, very still, eyes downcast. By the side of my plate my birthday present, a tin of Dobie's Blue Square tobacco, and next to it a long envelope. I didn't have to ask what it contained.

I had been expecting it for some time but it still gave me a jolt to find I had only a week before presenting myself at Lord's Cricket Ground, St John's Wood, London. And that week went by at frightening speed as I made my final plans, tidying up the loose ends in the practice, getting my Ministry of Agriculture forms sent off, arranging for our few possessions to be taken to Helen's old home where she would stay while I was away.

Having decided that I would finish work at teatime on Friday I had a call from old Arnold Summergill at about three o'clock that afternoon; and I knew that would be my very last job because it was always an expedition rather than a visit to his smallholding which clung to a bracken strewn slope in the depths of the hills. I didn't speak directly to Arnold but to Miss Thompson the postmistress in Hainby village.

'Mr Summergill wants you to come and see his dog,' she said over the phone.

'What's the trouble?' I asked.

I heard a muttered consultation at the far end.

'He says its leg's gone funny.'

'Funny? What d'you mean, funny?'

Again the quick babble of voices. 'He says it's kind of stickin' out.'

'All right,' I said. 'I'll be along very soon.'

It was no good asking for the dog to be brought in. Arnold had never owned a car. Nor had he ever spoken on a telephone – all our conversations had been carried on through the medium of Miss Thompson. Arnold would mount his rusty bicycle, pedal to Hainby and tell his troubles to the postmistress. And the symptoms; they were typically vague and I didn't suppose there would be anything either 'funny' or 'sticking out' about that leg when I saw it.

Anyway, I thought, as I drove out of Darrowby, I wouldn't mind having a last look at Benjamin. It was a fanciful name for a small farmer's dog and I never really found out how he had acquired it. But after all he was an unlikely breed for such a setting, a massive Old English Sheep Dog who would have looked more in place decorating the lawns of a stately home than following his master round Arnold's stony pastures. He was a classical example of the walking hearthrug and it took a second look to decide which end of him was which. But when you did manage to locate his head you found two of the most benevolent eyes imaginable glinting through the thick fringe of hair.

Benjamin was in fact too friendly at times, especially in winter when he had been strolling in the farmyard mud and showed his delight at my arrival by planting his huge feet on my chest. He did the same thing to my car, too, usually just after I had washed it, smearing clay lavishly over windows and bodywork while exchanging pleasantries with Sam inside. When Benjamin made a mess of anything he did it right.

But I had to interrupt my musings when I reached the last stage of my journey. And as I hung on to the kicking, jerking wheel and listened to the creaking and groaning of springs and shock absorbers, the thought forced its way into my mind as it always did around here that it cost us money to come to Mr Summergill's farm. There could be no profit from the visit because this vicious track must knock at least five pounds off the value of the car on every trip. Since Arnold did not have a car himself he saw no reason why he should interfere with the primeval state of his road.

It was simply a six foot strip of earth and rock and it wound and twisted for an awful long way. The trouble was that to get to the farm you had to descend into a deep valley before climbing through a wood towards the house. I think going down was worse because the vehicle hovered agonisingly on the top of each ridge before plunging into the yawning ruts beyond; and each time, listening to the unyielding stone grating on sump and exhaust I tried to stop myself working out the damage in pounds shillings and pence.

And when at last, mouth gaping, eyes popping, tyres sending the sharp pebbles flying, I ground my way upwards in bottom gear over the last few yards leading to the house I was surprised to see Arnold waiting for me there alone. It was unusual to see him without Benjamin.

He must have read my questioning look because he jerked his thumb over his shoulder.

'He's in t'house,' he grunted, and his eyes were anxious.

I got out of the car and looked at him for a moment as he stood there in a typical attitude, wide shoulders back, head high. I have called him 'old' and indeed he was over seventy, but the features beneath the woollen tammy which he always wore pulled down over his ears were clean and regular and the tall figure lean and straight. He was a fine looking man and must have been handsome in his youth, yet he had never married. I often felt there was a story there but he seemed content to live here alone, a 'bit of a 'ermit' as they said in the village. Alone, that is, except for Benjamin.

As I followed him into the kitchen he casually shooed out a couple of hens who had been perching on a dusty dresser. Then I saw Benjamin and pulled up with a jerk.

The big dog was sitting quite motionless by the side of the table and this time the eyes behind the overhanging hair were big and liquid with fright. He appeared to be too terrified to move and when I saw his left fore leg I couldn't blame him. Arnold had been right after all; it was indeed sticking out with a vengeance, at an angle which made my heart give a quick double thud; a complete lateral dislocation of the elbow, the radius projecting away out from the humerus at an almost impossible obliquity.

I swallowed carefully. 'When did this happen, Mr Summergill?'

'Just an hour since.' He tugged worriedly at his strange headgear. 'I was changing the cows into another field and awd Benjamin likes to have a nip at their heels when he's behind 'em. Well he did it once ower often and one of them lashed out and got 'im on the leg.'

'I see.' My mind was racing. This thing was grotesque. I had never seen anything like it, in fact thirty years later I still haven't seen anything like it. How on earth was I going to reduce the thing away up here in the hills ? By the look of it I would need general anaesthesia and a skilled assistant.

'Poor old lad,' I said, resting my hand on the shaggy head as I tried to think. 'What are we going to do with you ?'

The tail whisked along the flags in reply and the mouth

247

opened in a nervous panting, giving a glimpse of flawlessly white teeth.

Arnold cleared his throat. 'Can you put 'im right?'

Well it was a good question. An airy answer might give the wrong impression yet I didn't want to worry him with my doubts. It would be a mammoth task to get the enormous dog down to Darrowby; he nearly filled the kitchen, never mind my little car. And with that leg sticking out and with Sam already in residence. And would I be able to get the joint back in place when I got there? And even if I did manage it I would still have to bring him all the way back up here. It would just about take care of the rest of the day.

Gently I passed my fingers over the dislocated joint and searched my memory for details of the anatomy of the elbow. For the leg to be in this position the processus anconeus must have been completely disengaged from the supracondyloid fossa where it normally lay; and to get it back the joint would have to be flexed until the anconeus was clear of the epicondyles.

'Now let's see,' I murmured to myself. 'If I had this dog anaesthetised and on the table I would have to get hold of him like this.' I grasped the leg just above the elbow and began to move the radius slowly upwards. Benjamin gave me a quick glance then turned his head away, a gesture typical of good-natured dogs, conveying the message that he was going to put up with whatever I thought it necessary to do.

I flexed the joint still further until I was sure the anconeus was clear, then carefully rotated the radius and ulna inwards.

'Yes . . . yes . . .' I muttered again. 'This must be about the right position . . .' But my soliloquy was interrupted by a sudden movement of the bones under my hand; a springing, flicking sensation.

I looked incredulously at the leg. It was perfectly straight.

Benjamin, too, seemed unable to take it in right away, because he peered cautiously round through his shaggy curtain before lowering his nose and sniffing around the elbow. Then he seemed to realise all was well and ambled over to his master.

And he was perfectly sound. Not a trace of a limp.

A slow smile spread over Arnold's face. 'You've mended him, then.'

'Looks like it, Mr Summergill.' I tried to keep my voice casual, but I felt like cheering or bursting into hysterical laughter. I had only been making an examination, feeling things out a little, and the joint had popped back into place. A glorious accident.

'Aye well, that's grand,' the farmer said. 'Isn't it, awd lad?' He bent and tickled Benjamin's ear.

I could have been disappointed by this laconic reception of my performance, but I realised it was a compliment to me that he wasn't surprised that I, James Herriot, his vet, should effortlessly produce a miracle when it was required.

A theatre-full of cheering students would have rounded off the incident or it would be nice to do this kind of thing to some millionaire's animal in a crowded drawing room, but it never happened that way. I looked around the kitchen, at the cluttered table, the pile of unwashed crockery in the sink, a couple of Arnold's ragged shirts drying before the fire, and I smiled to myself. This was the sort of setting in which I usually pulled off my spectacular cures. The only spectators here, apart from Arnold, were the two hens who had made their way back on to the dresser and they didn't seem particularly impressed.

'Well, I'll be getting back down the hill,' I said. And Arnold walked with me across the yard to the car.

'I hear you're off to join up,' he said as I put my hand on the door.

'Yes, I'm away tomorrow, Mr Summergill.'

'Tomorrow, eh?' he raised his eyebrows.

'Yes, to London. Ever been there?'

'Nay, nay, be damned!' The woollen cap quivered as he shook his head. 'That'd be no good to me.'

I laughed. 'Why do you say that?'

'Well now, I'll tell ye.' He scratched his chin ruminatively. 'Ah nobbut went once to Brawton and that was enough. Ah couldn't walk on t'street!'

'Couldn't walk?'

'Nay. There were that many people about. I 'ad to take big steps and little 'uns, then big steps and little 'uns again. Couldn't get goin'.'

I had often seen Arnold stalking over his fields with the long, even stride of the hillman with nothing in his way and I knew exactly what he meant. 'Big steps and little 'uns.' That put it perfectly.

I started the engine and waved and as I moved away the old man raised a hand.

'Tek care, lad,' he murmured.

I spotted Benjamin's nose just peeping round the kitchen door. Any other time he would have been out with his master to see me off the premises but it had been a strange day for him culminating with my descending on him and mauling his leg about. He wasn't taking any more chances.

I drove gingerly down through the wood and before starting up the track on the other side I stopped the car and got out with Sam leaping eagerly after me.

This was a little lost valley in the hills, a green cleft cut off from the wild country above. One of the bonuses in a country vet's life is that he sees these hidden places. Apart from old Arnold nobody ever came down here, not even the postman who left the infrequent mail in a box at the top of the track and nobody saw the blazing scarlets and golds of the autumn trees nor heard the busy clucking and murmuring of the beck among its clean-washed stones.

I walked along the water's edge watching the little fish darting and flitting in the cool depths. In the spring these banks were bright with primroses and in May a great sea of bluebells flowed among the trees but today, though, the sky was an untroubled blue and the clean air was touched with the sweetness of the dying year.

I climbed a little way up the hillside and sat down among the bracken now fast turning to bronze. Sam, as was his way, flopped by my side and I ran a hand over the silky hair of his ears. The far side of the valley rose steeply to where, above the gleaming ridge of limestone cliffs, I could just see the sunlit rim of the moor.

I looked back to where the farm chimney sent a thin tendril of smoke from behind the brow of the hill, and it seemed that the episode with Benjamin, my last job in veterinary practice before I left Darrowby, was a fitting epilogue. A little triumph, intensely satisfying but by no means world shaking; like all the other little triumphs and disasters which make up a veterinary surgeon's life but go unnoticed by the world.

Last night, after Helen had packed my bag I had pushed Black's Veterinary Dictionary in among the shirts and socks. It was a bulky volume but I had been gripped momentarily by a fear that I might forget the things I had learned, and conceived on an impulse the scheme of reading a page or two each day to keep my memory fresh. And here among the bracken the thought came back to me; that it was the greatest good fortune not only to be fascinated by animals but to know about them. Suddenly the knowing became a precious thing.

I went back and opened the car door. Sam jumped on to the seat and before I got in I looked away down in the other direction from the house to the valley's mouth where the hills parted to give a glimpse of the plain below. And the endless wash of pale tints, the gold of the stubble, the dark smudges of wood, the mottled greens of the pasture land were like a perfect water colour. I found myself staring greedily as if for the first time at the scene which had so often lifted my heart, the great wide clean-blown face of Yorkshire.

I would come back to it all, I thought as I drove away; back to my work . . . how was it that book had described it . . . my hard, honest and fine profession.

I had to catch the early train and Bob Cooper was at the door with his ancient taxi before eight o'clock next morning.

Sam followed me across the room expectantly as he always did but I closed the door gently against his puzzled face. Clattering down the long flight of stairs I caught a glimpse through the landing window of the garden with the sunshine beginning to pierce the autumn mist, turning the dewy grass into a glittering coverlet, glinting on the bright colours of the apples and the last roses.

In the passage I paused at the side door where I had started my day's work so many times since coming to Darrowby, but then I hurried past. This was one time I went out the front.

Bob pushed open the taxi door and I threw my bag in before looking up over the ivy-covered brick of the old house to our little room under the tiles. Helen was in the window. She was crying. When she saw me she waved gaily and smiled, but it was a twisted smile as the tears flowed. And as we drove round the corner and I swallowed the biggest ever lump in my throat a fierce resolve welled in me; men all over the country were leaving their wives and I had to leave Helen now, but nothing, nothing, nothing would ever get me away from her again.

The shops were still closed and nothing stirred in the market place. As we left I turned and looked back at the cobbled square with the old clock tower and the row of irregular roofs with the green fells quiet and peaceful behind, and it seemed that I was losing something for ever.

I wish I had known then that it was not the end of everything. I wish I had known it was only the beginning. But at that moment I knew only that soon I would be far from here; in London, pushing my way through the crowds. Taking big steps and little 'uns.